BREAST
ULTRASOUND

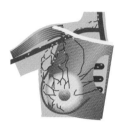

BREAST ULTRASOUND

Dr. M. E. Lanfranchi, M.D.

Professor of Ultrasound
The Argentine Society of Ultrasound in Medicine and Biology.
The Latin American Federation of Societies of Ultrasound in Medicine and Biology.
Chief, Section of Ultrasonography, Dr. A. Duhau Hospital.

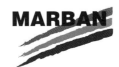

© 2000. **MARBAN BOOKS**, NY, NY
www.marban.com

ISBN 84-7101-247-2

Europe and Latin America
© **MARBÁN LIBROS, S.L.**
Joaquín María López, 72
28015 Madrid, Spain

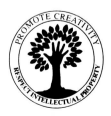

ISBN: 84-7101-247-2
M.33017.99
Printed in Spain

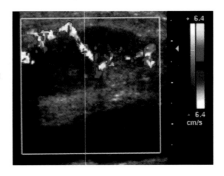

Dr. Mirta E. Lanfranchi, M.D.
Professor of Ultrasound
The Argentine Society of Ultrasound.
The Latin American Federation
of Ultrasound in Medicine and Biology.
Chief, Section of Ultrasonography, Dr. A. Duhau Hospital.

Co-author, chapter concerning color flow Doppler imaging:

Dr. Norman Koremblit, M.D.
President, International Chapter of the AIUM,
Argentine Ultrasound Group.
President Elect of the Latin-American Federation
of Ultrasound Societies.

Co-author, chapter on ultrasound guided intervention:

Dr. Roman Rostagno, M.D.
President, Society of Specialists in Mammary Pathologies.
Argentine Medical Foundation.

Technical Advisors:

Dr. Beatriz Cabeza , M.D.
Department of Radiology,
San Carlos Clinical Hospital
Madrid, Spain.

Paul Drevenstedt, B.A.
Georgia State University
Atlanta, Georgia, U.S.A.

Technical Supervision:

Dr. Jeff Allen, M.D.
Assistant Profesor of Radiology,
Emory University,
Atlanta, Georgia, U.S.A.

Dr. Craig Dick, M.D.
Emory University Affiliated Hospitals,
Atlanta, Georgia, U.S.A.

I give thanks for the life I have led
which has been so full....

To my parents, for allowing me to choose my own path,
and for supporting me with their love and care.

To my children, Silvina and Pablo, and my husband, Norman,
for understanding my absences and periods of silence while preparing this book.

And to my family and friends, for their patience and encouragement.

Preface

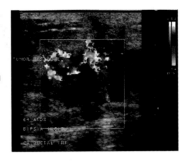

During the past ten years diagnostic ultrasound has been one of the fastest growing fields in medicine, thanks to constant advances in technology and the development of new techniques which take advantage of these advances. High definition and high frequency ultrasound allow the visualization of previously undetectable pathologies, making early diagnosis possible even in cases of non-palpable nodules. Color Doppler and Power Doppler permit the specialist to locate and study vascular signals in tumors, and three-dimensional ultrasound (3DUS) provides a representation of an object in three dimensions which is stored in computer memory and can be manipulated at will. Finally, but not least importantly, ultrasound-guided diagnostic intervention makes safer and more thorough the collection of cytological and histological samples.

The combination of ultrasound and mammography provides the specialist great diagnostic flexibility, as ultrasound is effective in cases where mammography is inappropriate, such as the differential diagnosis of pathologies in the radiologically dense breast, or other situations in which mammography proves inconclusive. This diagnostic flexibility translates to more effective medical care for the patient, especially in patients with breast cancer, a disease which affects as many as one out of every eight women and is often fatal if not detected early.

A well-trained ultrasound technologist and quality equipment are the two fundamental elements necessary for a successful ultrasound diagnosis. This book is intended to provide concrete examples of both rare and commonly encountered breast pathologies, and an outline of the techniques and technologies which are currently being used in the field. It is the hope of the authors and collaborators that this work will prove to be a valuable aid for the specialist and will contribute to the early and reliable diagnosis of breast pathologies.

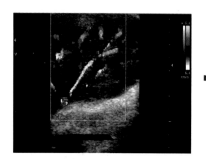

Table of Contents

Chapter **1**

Anatomy of the Breast
Topographical Anatomy of the Breast 13
Histoanatomy 14
Vascular Anatomy 18
Lymph Nodes 21
Sagittal Anatomical Images 22
Variations in the Breast 24

Chapter **2**

Equipment and Technique
Equipment 31
Ultrasound Examination Sequence 32

Chapter **3**

Simple and Complex Cyst Pathology
Introduction 39
Simple Cysts 40
Complex Cysts 47

Chapter **4**

Solid Benign Nodule
Fibroadenoma 57
Phyllodes Tumor 70
Papillomatosis 73
Nipple Adenoma 73
Benign Soft Tissue Tumors of the Breast 74
Other Benign Tumors 79

Chapter **5**

Solid Malignant Nodule
Introduction 83
Ultrasound in Nodules Undetectable by Mammography 85
WHO Classification 86
Malignant Nodules 88

Table of Contents

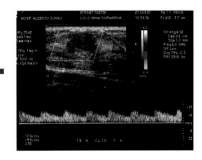

Chapter **6**

Diffuse Pathology of the Breast

Introduction	125
Pathological Stages of Fibrocystic Disease	125
Presence of Nodules	126
Classification of Ultrasound Images of FCD	126
Benign Lesions Associated with FCD	130
Dysplasia and Cancer	130
Diabetic Mastopathy	130

Chapter **7**

Ultrasound Examination of the Lactiferous Ducts   133

Chapter **8**

Trauma and Infections

Introduction	153
Mastitis	156

Chapter **9**

Ultrasound of Mammary Prostheses

Introduction	163
Evaluation of the Breast with Prosthesis	163
Complications from the Use of Implants	166
Complications in the Implant Itself	167
Evaluation of the Parenchyma in Patients with Implants	172
Injection of Free Silicone	174

Chapter **10**

Sequelae and Recurrence in the Breast Treated for Cancer

Introduction	177
Examination Outline	177
Benign Lesions	178
Statistics	186
Malignant Lesions	187

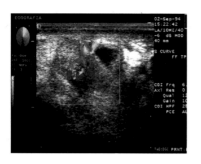

Table of Contents

Chapter **11**

Ultrasound-Guided Intervention

Introduction   193
Types of Intervention   197

Chapter **12**

Artifacts and Errors   215

Chapter **13**

Ultrasound in Post-Menopausal Women

Introduction   227
Common Pathologies   227
Post-Menopausal Breast Carcinoma   230

Chapter **14**

Color Doppler and Related Technologies

Introduction   231
Advantages and Limitations of Color Doppler   232
Advantages and Limitations of Amplitude/Energy Doppler   232
Invasive Ductal Carcinoma   239
Dynamic Angiographic Ultrasound (DAU 3D)   253
Lymph Node Evaluation with Color Doppler   260
Prognostic Possibilities   263
Evaluation of Auxillary Treatments   264
Angiostatic Agents   264
Contrast Agents   265

Chapter **15**

Three-Dimensional Ultrasound

Acquisition   274
Visualization   274

BREAST ULTRASOUND

1

Anatomy of the Breast

M. E. Lanfranchi

Topographical Anatomy of the Breast

The breast lies on the chest wall extending from the second to the sixth rib arch, and from the midline of the sternum to the midaxillary line.

Deep to the gland lies the pectoralis major, which runs from the clavicle to the sternum, and from the rib arches to the upper part of the anterolateral region of the humerus.

Subadjacent to the pectoralis major the pectoralis minor is found, which extends from the third to the fifth rib, and up to the coracoid apophysis of the scapula.

The inferolateral aspect of the gland lies on the serratus anterior muscle. The entire gland is contained within the superficial layers and the deep layers of the superficial fascia of the pectoralis major.

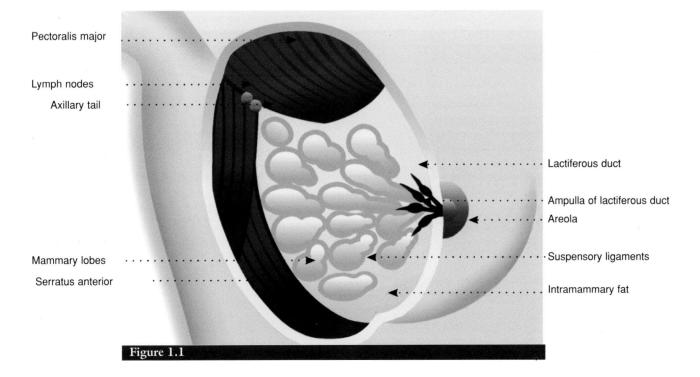

Pectoralis major

Lymph nodes

Axillary tail

Lactiferous duct

Ampulla of lactiferous duct

Areola

Mammary lobes

Serratus anterior

Suspensory ligaments

Intramammary fat

Figure 1.1

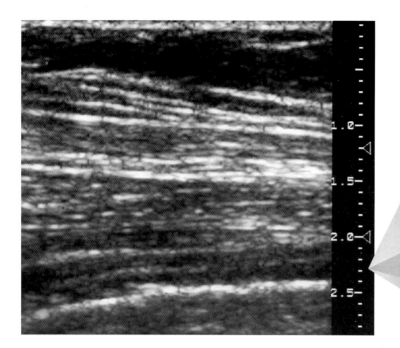

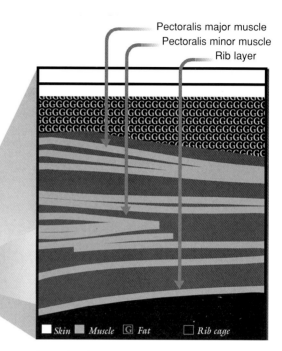

Fig. 1.2 Characteristic appearance of pectoral muscles in a longitudinal section: multiple lineal images ("laminates") of varying echogenicity.

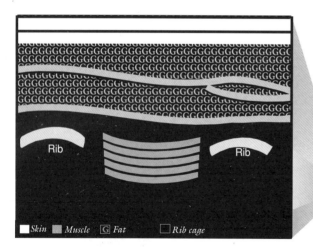

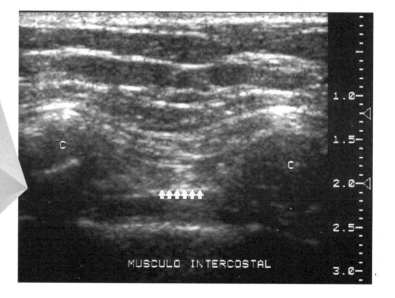

Fig. 1.3 Transverse section of the plane of the ribs showing, from the surface to the interior: skin and intramammary fat. Transverse section of two ribs (hypoechoic image with posterior acoustic shadow) and intercostal muscle (laminate appearance).

Histoanatomy

The mammary crest develops during the fourth week of fetal development from ectodermical tissue. It determines the mammary ridge, which extends from the axilla to the inguinal region. Due to various transformations of the adipose and epithelial precursors, it will give rise to the primary breasts, which in the third trimester of pregnancy are influenced by the action of hormones such as estrogen, progesterone and prolactine.

Accessory nipples and/or ectopic glandular tissue may be found on any point of the mammary ridge or the axilla when there are disorders in the initial stages of embryological development.

Anomalies such as the asymmetrical development of the breasts, or less frequently, amastia, can also occur.

After birth and development the breast is found between the two layers of the superficial fascia of the pectoralis major. Between the two layers the internal structures of the breast are supported by suspensory ligaments (Cooper's ligaments).

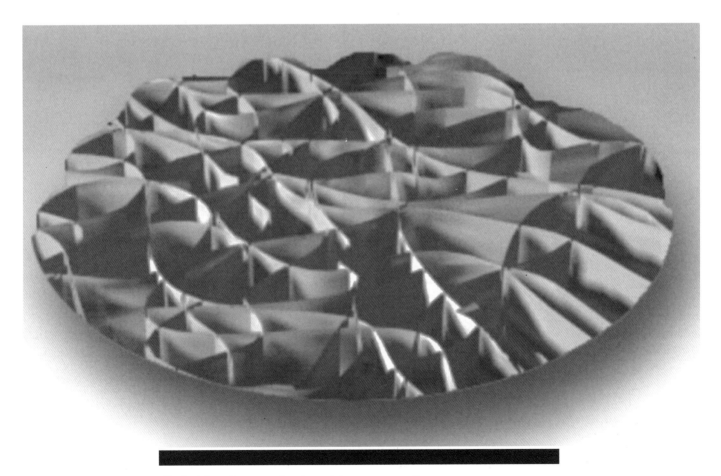

Fig 1.4 Anterior-posterior view of the suspensory ligaments.

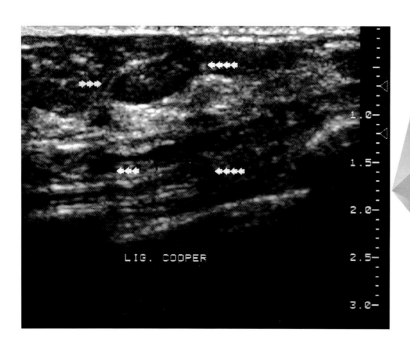

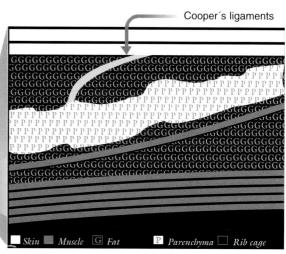

Fig. 1.5 The Cooper's ligaments appear as linear echogenic images which pass through the cellular tissue in the direction of the skin. From the surface to the interior the following can be distinguished: skin, superficial fascia, glandular tissue, retromammary fat, muscle layer, and rib layer.

The gland is composed of glandular tissue and supported by fibrous connective tissue. The glandular tissue consists of approximately 15 to 20 lobes, each connected to a particular lactiferous duct. Each lactiferous duct divides beneath the areola and branches into smaller ducts.

A number of the lactiferous ducts terminate abruptly a few centimeters from the nipple, while others branch in order to drain different sectors of the breast.

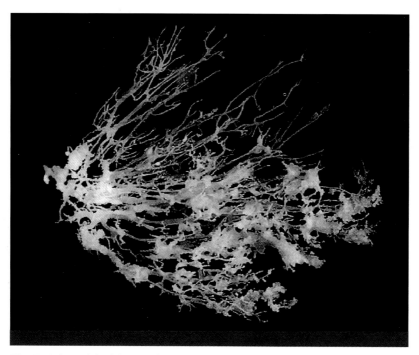

Fig. 1.6 A model of the lactiferous ducts and ampullas. The areolar region is to the left, with large principal ducts and smaller secondary ducts.

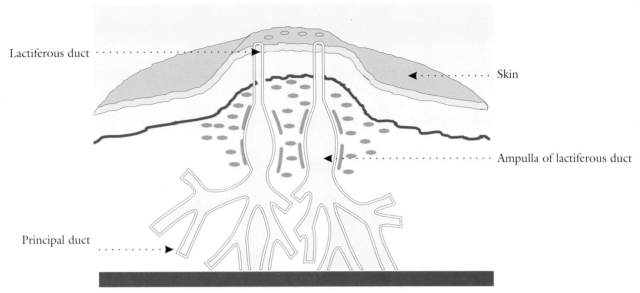

Fig 1.7 In the nipple there are approximately 20 lactiferous duct openings. Each opening leads to a lactiferous sinus and then to the principal ducts.

The areola is the pigmented area which surrounds the nipple, and it contains sebaceous and areolar glands (of Montgomery), which lubricate the area during lactation. The areolar glands may also secrete milk as accessory glands.

The nipple is composed of stratified squamous epithelium, dense collagenic tissue, and small muscles which are interrupted by the openings of the lactiferous ducts. These ducts terminate in glandular cul-de-sacs and have two parts: the extralobular, which stems from intralobular branches, and the intralobular, which is terminal and surrounds the acini.

The connective tissue of the stroma surrounds and separates the ductal components from the lobular elements.

The stroma which surrounds the ducts is composed of cells and contains blood and lymph vessels. Therefore, even in normal circumstances it is possible to find a small lymph node, especially in the upper-external quadrant of the breast.

The deepest portion of the breast lies on top of a layer of adipose tissue (the retroglandular fatty layer).

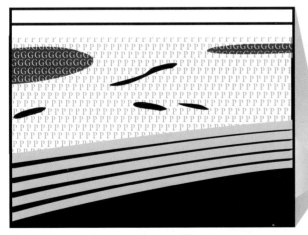

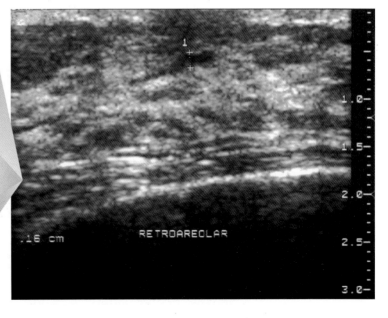

Fig. 1.8 Image of a normal breast. The skin appears as two echogenic lines with a central hypoechoic area. The gland is of medium echogenicity while the tubular-type lactiferous ducts are anechoic. The superficial fascia and the retromammary band are both hypoechoic and can be seen, as well as the muscle layer (laminate appearance) and the rib layer (hyperechogenic line).

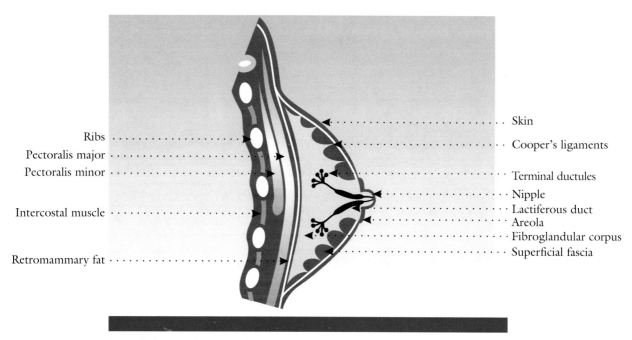

Fig 1.9 A sagittal section of the breast by layers.

Vascular Anatomy

Blood is supplied to the breast by branches of the axillary artery, the external mammary artery, the internal mammary artery (or internal thoracic), and the intercostal arteries.

The lateral and deep portions of the breast are supplied by the external and intercostal mammary arteries, and the medial portion is supplied by branches of the internal mammary artery.

The superior thoracic artery originates in the first portion of the axillary artery and supplies the pectoralis major and the deep part of the gland.

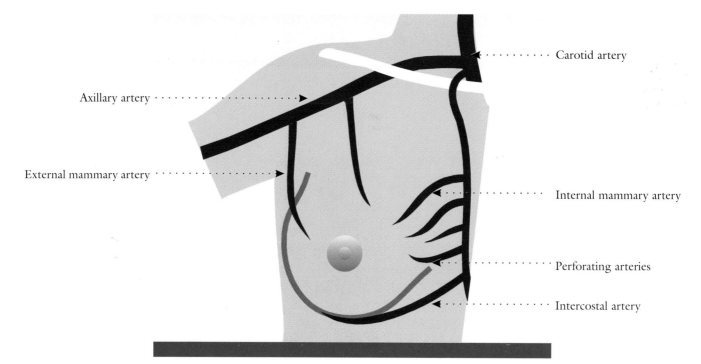

Fig 1.10 The breast is supplied blood mainly by the internal and external mammary arteries, and to a lesser degree by the intercostal and perforating arteries.

The achromioclavicular artery and the lateral thoracic artery originate from the second portion of the axillary artery, coursing between and supplying both pectoralis muscles. The lateral thoracic artery runs along the edge of the pectoralis major and supplies the lateral portion of the breast, which is also supplied blood by branches of the subscapular artery.

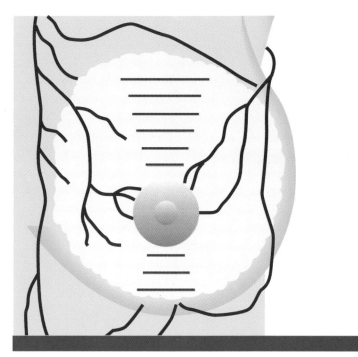

Fig 1.11 Diagram of the safe areas (=) linked to the principal vascular pedicles. The areas indicated by the lines are free of major veins and arteries, and thus are of clinical relevance.

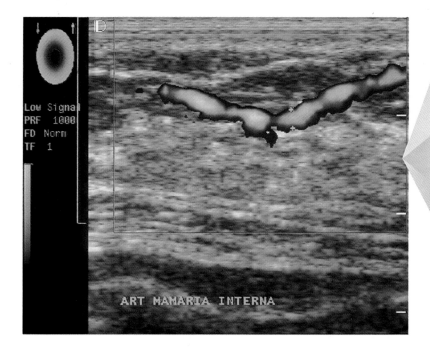

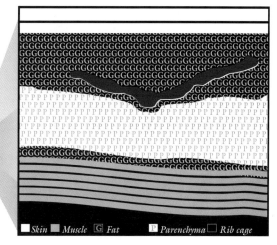

☐ *Skin* ☐ *Muscle* G *Fat* P *Parenchyma* ☐ *Rib cage*

Fig. 1.12 The internal mammary artery located along the edge of the gland.

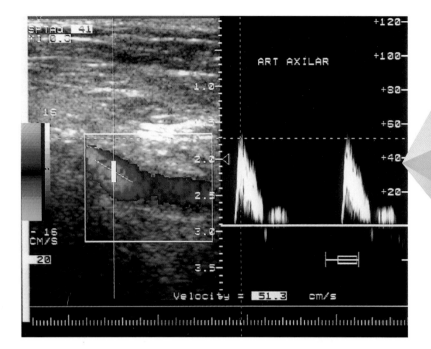

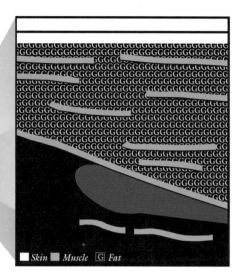

Fig. 1.13 The axillary artery located within the tissues of the axilla. The diameter of the artery in this image ranges from 5 to 8 mm and displays normal blood flow.

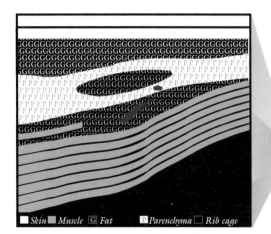

Fig. 1.14 A branch of the external mammary artery located in the glandular tissue of the upper-outer quadrant.

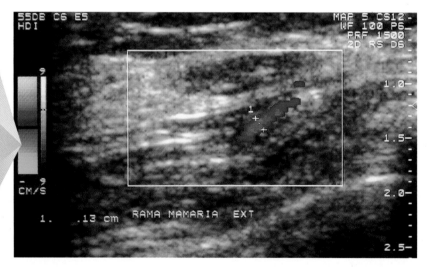

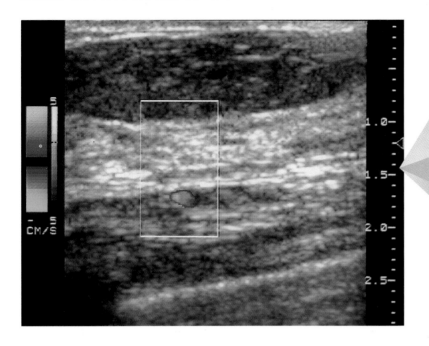

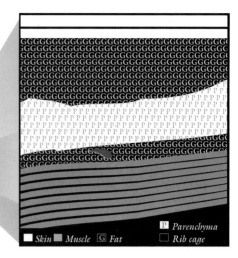

Fig. 1.15 A branch of the anterior perforating artery located in the retromammary fat between the muscle and the gland.

Lymph Nodes

The deep and subareolar lymph nodes join with the subareolar plexus and lead to different regions. The majority of the lymphatic drainage of the breast is carried out by the axillary lymph nodes, while the parasternal (sternal, internal mammary) and subcutaneous nodes are responsible for a smaller portion of the drainage.

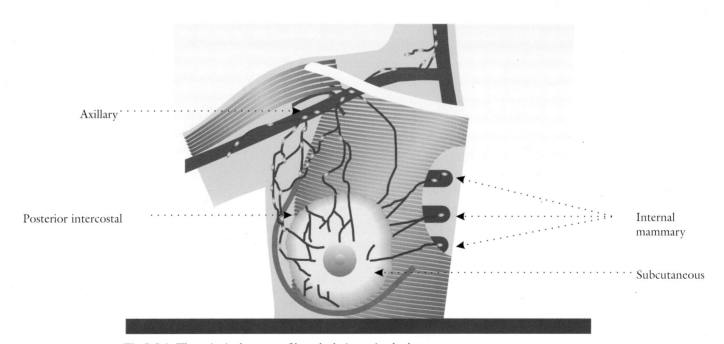

Fig 1.16 The principal routes of lymph drainage in the breast:

1) Pectoral axillary nodes   2) Apical axillary nodes
2) Parasternal nodes   4) Subcutaneous nodes

The axillary lymph nodes are divided into the following groups:

- **Subscapular nodes**
- **Pectoral nodes**
- **Interpectoral nodes**
- **Apical nodes**
- **Infraclavicular subgroup of nodes**

For surgical purposes, the axillary lymph nodes are divided into three groups or levels, according to their relation with the pectoralis minor:

- **Level I:** lateral in relation to the pectoralis minor
- **Level II:** deep to the pectoralis minor
- **Level III:** between the medial border of the pectoralis minor and the first rib.

The flow of lymph in the breast follows the path of the lymph vessels in the fatty tissues overlying the intercostal muscles. In the upper region, including the third intercostal space, the lymph nodes correspond with the parietal pleura, but in the distal region, they correspond with the internal mammary vessels and are 3 cm away from the sternal edge.

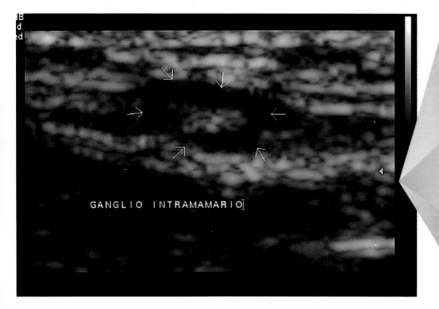

GANGLIO INTRAMAMARIO

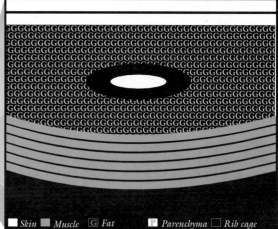

□ *Skin* ■ *Muscle* G *Fat* P *Parenchyma* □ *Rib cage*

Fig. 1.17 Image of a normal lymph node: a hyperechogenic center (hila) surrounded by hyperechoic tissue (the lymph node itself).

Sagittal Anatomical Images

Between the surface and the interior of the breast one finds the image which corresponds with the dermis and epidermis which compose the skin.

Using high frequency transducers (7.5 MHz or more) one observes two echogenic lines. These lines are interposed by a hypoechoic band of adipose tissue, which is the interphase between the two zones. Normally, the width of the skin is between 2 and 3mm, being somewhat thicker at the areola.

Between the mammary gland (surrounded by the superficial and deep layers of the superficial fascia of the pectoralis major) and the skin one finds a layer of hypoechoic adipose tissue of variable width.

The suspensory (or Cooper's) ligaments, which form the supporting structure between the superficial and deep leaves of the superficial fascia, are most clearly seen in involutive breasts with adipose infiltration. They appear as very thin hyperechogenic lines extending from the surface of the gland to the superficial fascia, and may present a posterior sonic shadow if the ultrasound beam strikes its own axis.

The mammary gland is composed of glandular tissue and is supported by fibrous connective tissue. It appears as a hyperechogenic image, whose homogenicity depends upon the interlobular stroma which is composed of fibroadipose tissue. Between the posterior surface of the gland and the pectoralis major (with deep fascia) one finds the retromammary space, which is occupied by retromammary hypoechoic adipose tissue.

The nipple and the tissue directly beneath it are the most difficult to evaluate by ultrasound because, depending on the technique employed, a shadow may be produced behind the nipple, preventing good definition in the image.

The muscle fibers, the large amount of connective tissue, and the nipple itself may be responsible for this difficulty. The image of the nipple may be round or oval and of medium echogenicity. In the subareolar region one may observe tubular hypoechoic or anechoic structures, which are the lactiferous ducts which converge at the nipple.

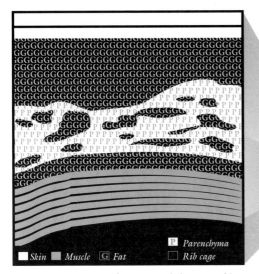

Fig. 1.18 Image of a normal breast: skin, superficial fascia, retromammary layer, and rib layer.

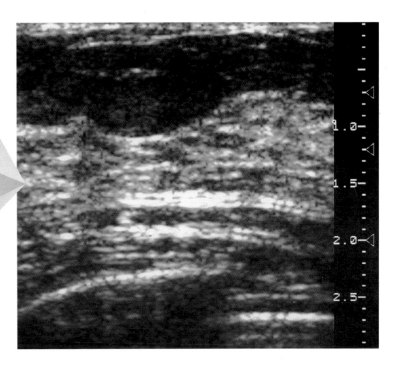

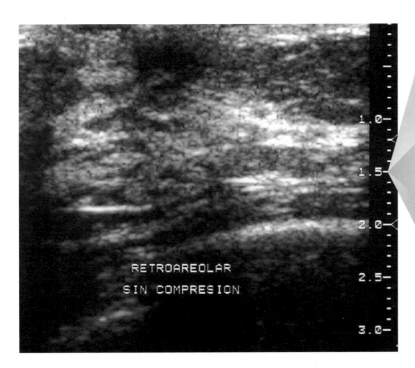

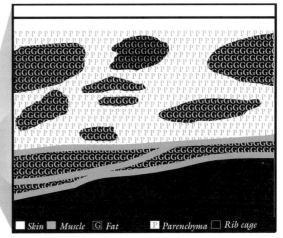

Fig. 1.19 Retroareolar region of a normal breast showing normal sonic attenuation in the center. The gland is heterogeneous and shows areas of adipose infiltration.

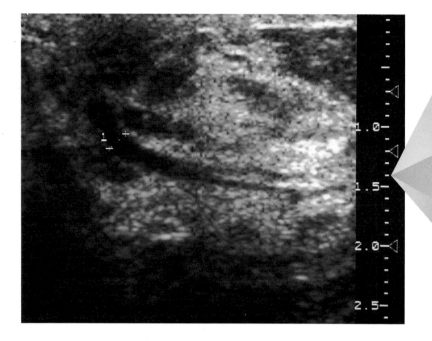

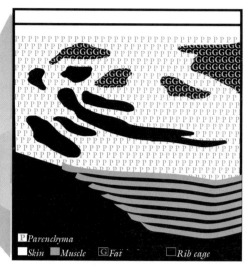

Fig 1.20 Retroareolar exploration of a normal breast. The central hypoechoic pseudonodular image is the nipple, upon which the tubular lactiferous ducts (echonegative) converge.

Variations in the Breast

1. The Breast During Childhood

The mammary button appears as a round or oval image, either hypoechoic or of medium echogenicity, which is in contact with the skin and is surrounded by a thin layer of fatty tissue.

Directly beneath the button lies the pectoralis major and the rib layer (which, when viewed in longitudinal or transverse section, may cause a posterior acoustic shadow). The image of the mammary button shows fibrous connective tissue in which no lobes have developed yet, and which contains a number of small lactiferous ducts.

The image will remain the same, except for variations in size according to physical characteristics, until one or two years before menarche. Then, rapid glandular growth takes place, mainly due to the hormonal action of estrogens. This growth is accompanied by the formation of lobes and an increase in the size and number of branches of the ducts.

Asymmetrical development of the glands during puberty is not uncommon and does not normally indicate a pathological condition.

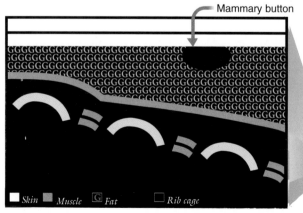

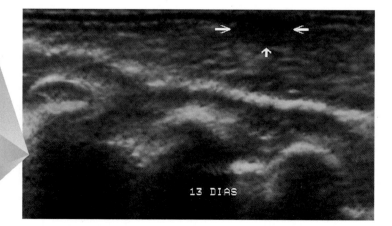

Fig. 1.21 Image of the mammary button of a 13 day-old girl.

2. The Adolescent Breast

During this period the gland occupies most of the breast and there is little intramammary and retromammary fat. The parenchyma reaches its full size and in sonograms generally appears hyperechogenic and homogeneous.

However, in some cases a normal variation occurs in which the parenchyma appears spotted (hyperechogenic with small hypoechoic areas).

In obese adolescents the mammary fat may produce heterogenous images with irregular hypoechoic areas.

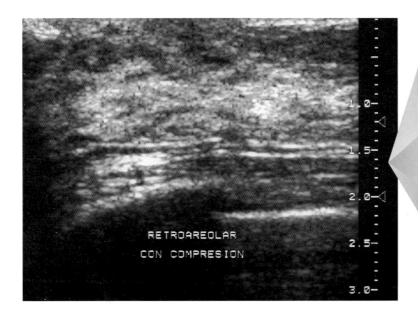

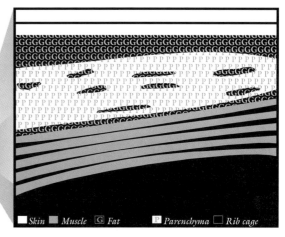

Fig. 1.22 Normal breast of an adolescent. Note the greater echogenicity of the gland.

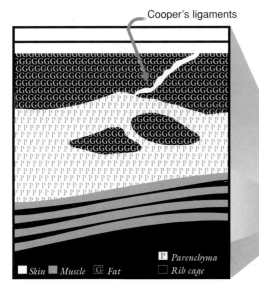

Fig. 1.23 Breast of an adolescent in which the mammary fat appears as hypoechoic areas.

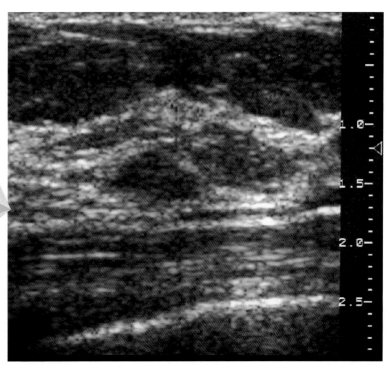

3. The Breast During Middle Age

The echostructure of the gland during this stage is generally heterogenous, with variations according to the density of the parenchyma and the amount of intramammary fat.

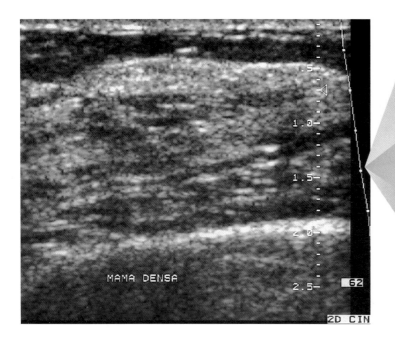

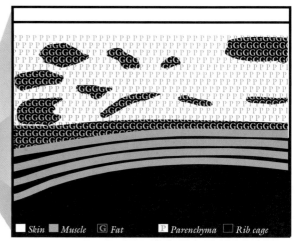

Fig. 1.24 Gland with a spotted appearance (due to intramammary fat) in a 30 year-old woman.

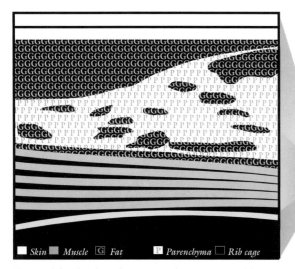

Fig. 1.25 Gland with a spotted appearance (due to intramammary fat) in a 40 year-old woman.

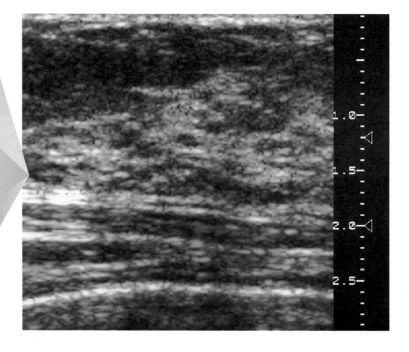

4. The Breast During Pregnancy and Lactation

During this period there is a significant increase in the size of the lobules, which displace the parenchyma. For this reason the glandular tissue appears homogeneous with an increase in echogenicity and the visualization of tubular structures (lactiferous ducts) is common.

During lactation the glandular image becomes finely granular and a series of dilated and prominent ducts (round or oval images) may be obseved. Although they appear to be cysts, they are actually the lactiferous ducts.

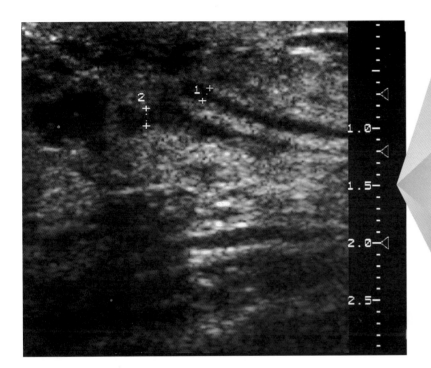

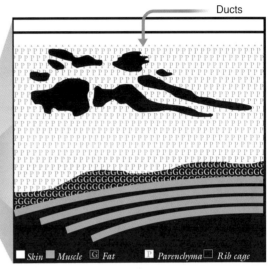

Fig. 1.26 Lactiferous ducts (anechoic) of normal size observed from the retroareolar region.

5. The Senile Breast

In post-menopausic women the majority of the parenchyma is replaced by fatty tissue. This process is progressive and in the elderly breast generally little glandular tissue remains.

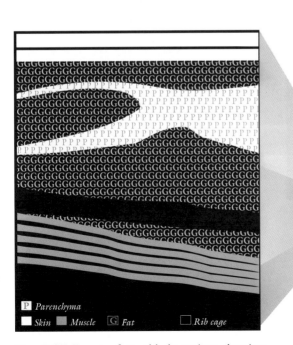

Fig. 1.27 Breast of an elderly patient showing abundant fatty tissue.

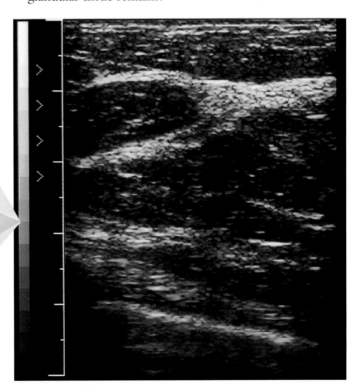

The preceding images have been separated and placed under five headings for didactic purposes. They are examples of the normal structural changes in the breast which one may observe using ultrasound.

By studying numerous images of normal breasts one becomes proficient at recognizing whether or not a sonogram is normal for the age group of the patient.

The breast, and hence the images of it, are dynamic. They may vary according to phases of the menstrual cycle, hormonal treatments, or the biological age of the patient.

The ability to diagnose pathologies of the breast comes only after one is thoroughly proficient at evaluating and recognizing normal breast ultrasound images. Therefore, it is fundamental that one be aware of and familiar with the range of variations which occur in normal breasts.

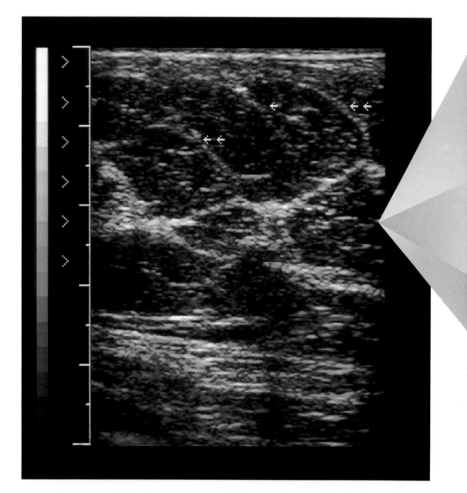

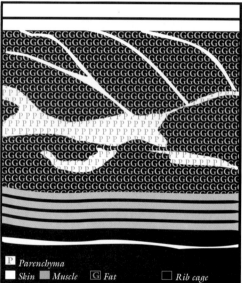

P Parenchyma
Skin   Muscle   G Fat   Rib cage

Fig. 1.28 Hypoechoic breast of an elderly patient with replacement of the parenchyma by fatty tissue.

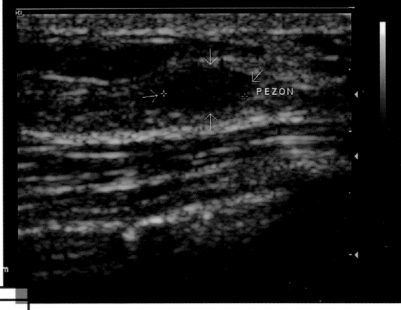

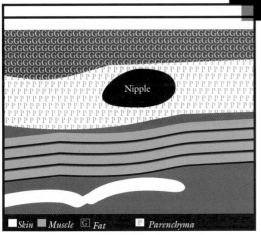

Fig. 1.29 Breast of a 24 year-old patient. When the transducer is placed over it the nipple will appear as a hypoechoic, homogeneous image with well-defined borders a few millimeters below the surface.

References

- Baset LW, Kimme-Smith C: Breast sonography: technique, equipment and normal anatomy. *Sem Ultrasound CTMR*, 1989; 10:82-89.
- Schenck CD, Lehman DA: Sonographic anatomy of the breast. *Smin Ultrasound*, 1982, 3:13-33.
- Hackson VP, Kelly-Fry E, Rothschild PA, Holden RW, Clark SA: Automated breast sonography using a 7,5 MHz PVDF transducer: preliminary clinical evaluation. *Radiology*, 1986; 159:679-684.

2

Equipment and Technique

M. E. Lanfranchi

Equipment

In order to perform good ultrasonic examinations of the breast it is necessary to have the proper equipment .

If it is to allow the doctor to detect lesions early or delimit small nodules the equipment must have:

-Linear transducers of 7.5 MHz, or higher frequency.

-Good space and contrast resolution.

-Good close field resolution and an optimum penetration of 4 cm.

The evolution of ultrasound technology and the improvement of materials have optimized diagnostic ultrasound, both improving the definition of images and reducing the noise effect (artifact).

High resolution allows us to distinguish small lesions from the rest of the parenchyma; the higher frequencies are used to demonstrate ductal anatomy or pathology.

The preference for lineal array transducers is easily understood by comparing the three different types of transducers and their respective focal zones.

■ Optimal focal zone

Lineal

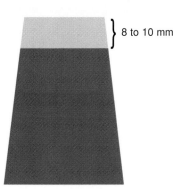

8 to 10 mm

Annular (electronic)

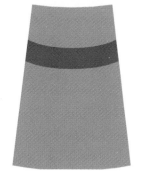

A sector of an element (mechanic)

Figure 2.1

Spatial resolution is a 3D measurement which consists of three components: axial, lateral and azimuth or elevation, and determines the ability of the equipment to differenciate two structures of similar echogenicity.

Axial resolution may be defined as the minimum separation between two points of tissue in a direction parallel to the ultrasound beam; as a result two distinct structures appear on the screen. The most important factor in determining the axial resolution is the pulse length. This is closely related to the frequency of the transducer; when the frequency is lowered penetration is augmented.

In order to overcome limitations in axial resolution the ceramic components in transducers were replaced by wide-band components, which allow the axial resolution to improve beyond the previous wavelength limits.

31

Lateral resolution is the ability to differenciate two objects which are close to one another and perpendicular to the ultrasound beam.

This is determined by the width of the ultrasound beam; lateral resolution is augmented by fine beams, and is maximized at the focal zone.

Lateral resolution is the major limiting factor of image quality. Artifacts which originate outside the focal zone are significant and can lead to incorrect diagnoses. For this reason a number of modifications to the original model have been made in order to improve lateral resolution.

The most important factor to consider when choosing a transducer should be the depth of the area of interest. Contrast resolution determines both the ability to distinguish the presence of tissues with small amplitude echoes adjacent to tissues with much larger echoes (high contrast resolution) and the ability to differentiate between tissues which have similar amplitude echoes (low contrast resolution). Both high and low contrast resolutions are due to the differences in the acoustic impedance of tissues.

The need for good spatial resolution in equipment which provides high resolution is widely recognized, especially in order to differentiate small lesions and ducts. But contrast resolution is the most important parameter which determines the ability to differentiate variations which occur in the pathological breast. Contrast resolution is dependent upon the characteristics of the transducers, the parameters of the signals processed, the background tissue, and the artifact.

The ultrasound beam is modified as it travels through different tissues, producing the phenomenon of attenuation. With increases in depth, attenuation increases while intensity decreases.

Attenuation results from the combination of the absorption, reflectivity, and diffusion of ultrasound.

Attenuation increases along with frequency; approximately 1 dB/cm/MHz in soft tissues.

The amplitude of a beam of 7.5 MHz is attenuated more than 50% for each centimeter of depth.

This loss can be corrected by augmenting the depth amplitude (TGC: time gain compensation), thus maintaining the correlation between the brilliance of the image and the intensity of the echo.

If a lesion absorbs more than the surrounding tissue for which the TGC has been adjusted, the deep tissue appears darker (hypoechoic). This is called shadow and usually appears in carcinomas.

On the other hand, when the echoes behind an attenuated lesion are overcompensated and appear more intense (hyperechogenic) than the surrounding tissue, the effect is called posterior acoustic enhancement, and usually appears in cysts.

In summary, good ultrasound equipment must have the following characteristics:
- **Matrix:** 512 x 512 x 8 bits.
- **Grey scale:** 256
- **Lateral:** 0.1 mm.
- **Axial:** 0.15 mm.
- **Optimun focalization zone:** from 0.2 to 4 cm (xcr 110-5).

Although the diagnostic use of breast ultrasound as a compliment to mammography is widely accepted, some specialists only use this method in circumscribed palpable lesions and doubtful mammographies. However, breast ultrasound may also be used to rule out lesions, a technique which requires good training and a detailed examination of the entire breast. This method is of considerable importance when one considers the fact that 25 to 30% of breast carcinomas occur in premenopausic women, in whom mammographical screening has shown certain limitations.

Ultrasound Examination Sequence

A breast ultrasound examination shoud be conducted in the following order:

1. **General questions:**
    - Reason for consulting the physician
    - Palpable or non-palpable pathology
    - Antecedents (surgery, trauma, lactation, silicone implants, discharges from the nipple, ect.)
2. **Mammography**
3. **Inspection:**
    - Asymmetries
    - Scars
    - Retractions or bulges

- Hematomas
- Signs of inflammation or infection
4. **Palpation:**
    - of the whole breast
    - of the areolar region
    - of the axila
5. **Thoroughly explain** the clinical findings and mark down on the skin when a nodule or an induration is encountered.
6. **Technique**
    The following must be considered:
    - Position of the patient
    - Exploration or scan mode

-Position of the transducer
-Exploration of:
-Parenchyma (identification of layers)
-Ductal system (with or without compression)
-Scars
-Handling and variations of the power gain
-Circular exploration of a lesion (borders)
7. **In case of a lesion, investigate:**
-Echogenicity
-Echostructure
-Mobility and compressibility
-Behavior of the surrounding tissues
-Behavior of the superficial fascia

-Behavior of the posterior tissues (enhancement or posterior acoustic shadow)
-Axillary exploration

By having the patient lie in a supine position with both hands placed by the sides or behind the head, the entire breast is extended along the pectoral muscle and the rib cage.

This position is optimal for evaluation of all quadrants and anatomical layers of the breast.

At this point in the examination three diferent types of ultrasound scans can be carried out (Fig. 2.2).

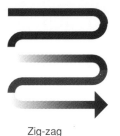
Zig-zag

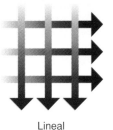
Lineal

Convergent

Figure 2.2

As ultrasound images are tomographic sections, if they are not correctly performed it is possible for small or non-palpable pathologies to pass unnoticed. Therefore, it is important to carry out a detailed exploration of all the quadrants of the breast. For this reason the first two metods, the zig-zag and the linear, are the most efficient.

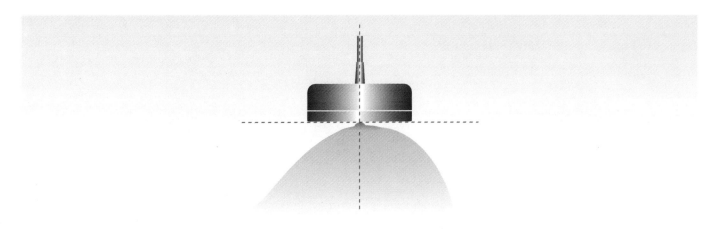

Figure 2.3

The transducer should always be perpendicular to the breast, in order to prevent false images or distortions.

The first scan should focus on recognition of the anatomical layers and the condition of the gland itself (see variations in Chapter I).

Once the scanning of the four quadrants of the gland (upper outer, upper inner, lower outer, lower inner) is complete, the areola and the nipple (where the lactiferous ducts are found) are evaluated.

There are two metods of positioning the transducer in order to explore this sector (Fig 2.4).

As stated in Chapter one, the exploration of this area may produce sonic attenuation, depending on the pressure applied by the operator.

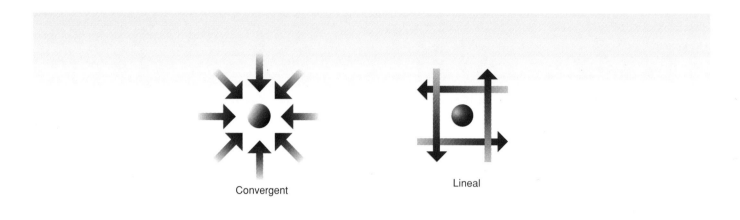

Convergent

Lineal

Figure 2.4

In cases in which the patient has experienced discharge from the nipple, a detailed evaluation of the lactiferous ducts should be performed. The ducts should be examined along their trajectory in both transverse and sagittal sections, in order to evaluate their walls and contents and rule out any dilation (a diameter greater than 4mm). When exploring a surgical scar, one should closely examine the modifications to the skin, the superficial fascia, and the parenchyma.

In recent scars there is generally a thickening of the skin (width greater than 2-3mm) caused by edema and a diffuse alteration of the echogenicity of the superficial fascia and the parenchyma.

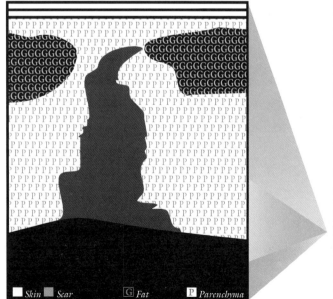

Skin Scar G Fat P Parenchyma

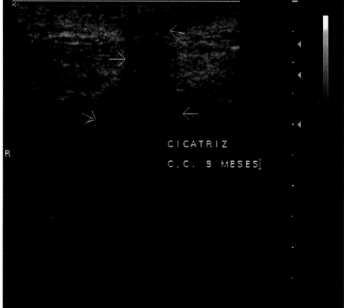

Fig. 2.5 Image taken 8 months after surgery showing thickening of the skin due to edema and discrete destruction of the tissues.

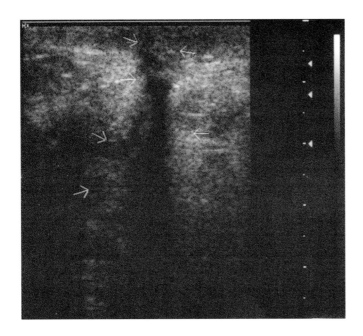

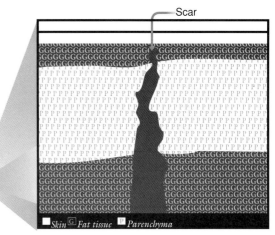

Fig. 2.6 Image taken 9 months after surgery of the right breast. The surgical scar shows fibrosis which begins at skin level and descends to the glandular level.

Under normal circumstances edema eventually disappears and gives way to fibrosis, which may produce sonic attenuation in ultrasound images.

The following equipment controls must be adjusted for any exploration focusing on a specific point in the breast:

- **Focalization or focus depth:** in order to optimize image definition.
- **Power gain curve:** in order to avoid artifacts or interpretation errors.
- **Brilliance and contrast:** in order to highlight the borders and contents.

This stage of examination is extremely important, as the correct diagnosis will depend on the following elements:

- **Adequate equipment**
- **The equipment operator's training**
- **The technique employed**

In cases where nodules are present, it is important that its contents and borders are properly evaluated.

In order to evaluate the border of a nodule circular technique may be applied, which consists of rotating the transducer 360 degrees on its axis, which facilitates insonation of the nodule's outline.

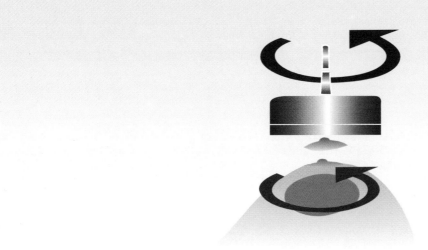

Circular technique

Figure 2.7

The mobility and compressibility of a nodule are generally good criteria to use in determining if it is benign.

Benign masses usually move aside or compress surrounding tissue, and produce clean, uniform, and homogeneous images. Malignant masses, on the other hand, infiltrate the tissue or display desmoplastic reactions, and produce heterogeneous and anarchic echos.

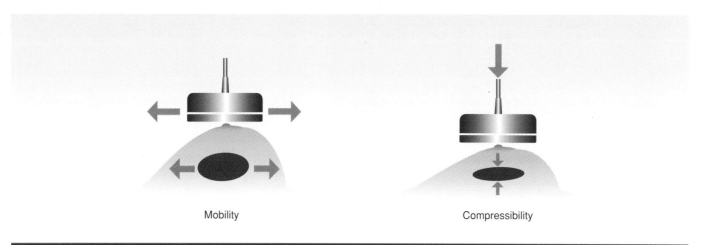

Mobility   Compressibility

Figure 2.8

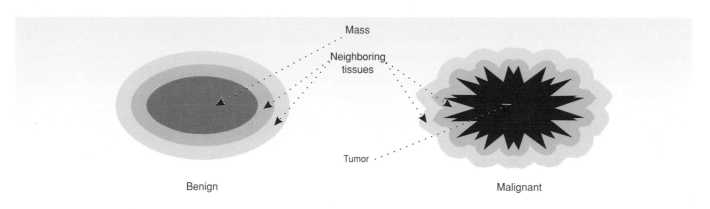

Mass

Neighboring tissues

Tumor

Benign   Malignant

Figure 2.9

There are a number of ways in which the superficial fascia may be altered in the presence of a tumor.

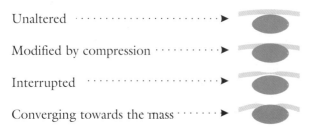

Unaltered

Modified by compression

Interrupted

Converging towards the mass

The two last cases generally observed in malignant tumors.

In general, the quality of the ultrasound image of a lesion depends on the following factors:

Size of the tumor
Echogenicity
Growth pattern
The surrounding tissues

When sonic attenuation is encountered there are two possible explanations. The first, explained on page 32, is that the attenuation is produced by the passage of the ultrasound beam through various tissues. This can be corrected by modifying the equipment's power gain curve.

The second possibility is that the attenuation is caused by the characteristics of the tissues. For this reason the following different diagnoses should be considered:

– Scar
– Fibrosis
– Retroareolar zone
– Rib layer
– Certain carcinomas

When a malignant tumor is suspected the axillary region shoud be investigated. In this region one may find either a normal lymph node or one suspected of metastatic infiltration (as we will see in Chapter 5).

During such investigations one should keep in mind the normal anatomy of the axillary region and its relation to the pectoralis major and minor.

A normal lymph node generally has an elongated shape and greater echogenicity at its center. This increased echogenicity is due to the hilum and its vascular and adipose components.

When the ultrasonic examination is concluded, a diagnostic report must be prepared, which includes two sections:

1. **Description of the lesion:**

    – Location
    – -Size
    – Echogenicity
    – Echostructure (solid or cystic)
    – Borders and limits
    – Characteristics of the posterior border (enhancement or attenuation)
    – Layers it affects
    – Mobility (and compressibility)
    – Behavior of the surrounding tissues
    – Does it correspond with the clinical examination and/or mammography?
    – Does it engage the lymph nodes?

2. **Diagnostic conclusion:**

    – Process compatible with...

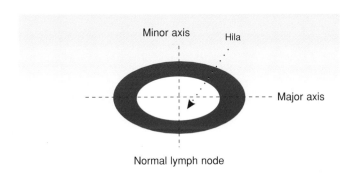

Figure 2.10

If a nodule is found it is helpful to plot its location graphically using a model similar to the following:

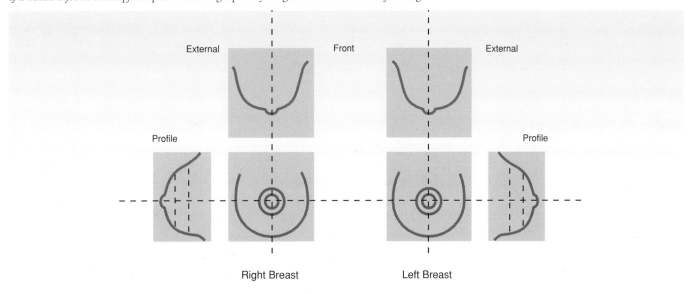

Figure 2.11

References

- Hermann G, Schwartz IS: Focal fibrous disease of the breast: Mammographic detection of an unappreciated condition. *AJR*, 1983; 140: 1245-1246.
- Egan: *Breast imaging, diagnosis and morphology of breast disease*. Philadelphia, Saunders, 1988, pp. 213-215.
- Gerson ES: Fibrocystic "disease" (letter). *Radiology*, 1988; 168: 421-423.
- Love SM, Gelman RS, Silen W: Fibrocystic "disease" of the breast - A non-disease? *N Engl J Med*, 1982; 307: 1010-1014.
- Harris JR, Hellman S, Henderson JC, Kinne DW: *Breast diseases*, ed. 2. Philadelphia, Lippincott, 1991, pp. 15-20.
- Consensus Meeting: Is "fibrocystic disease" of the breast precancerus? *Arch Pathol Lab Med*, 1986, 110: 171-173.

3

Simple and Complex Cyst Pathology

M. E. Lanfranchi

Introduction

Fibrocystic disease (FCD) is the oldest recognized pathology of the breast. The development of cysts is generally accompanied by numerous microscopic changes. Epithelial proliferation is predominant among these changes, and it may be accompanied by both atrophy and fibrosis.

The term "macrocystic disease" is used if the cysts in question are large or palpable, while the term "microcystic disease" is used if small or non-palpable cysts are present.

Fibrocystic disease is the most common lesion of the breast and constitutes approximately 25% of all nodes found by palpation and/or mammography. Statistically, one out of every six to eight women will develop this disease.

Macrocysts generally appear during middle age, although unitary unilateral lesions may be found in women as young as 20 years of age. Nevertheless, they most commonly appear between the ages of 35 and 50, and very rarely occur after menopause.

Close to 10% of women with FCD display antecedents of unilateral or bilateral palpable cysts. Once these cysts have appeared, new ones often develop at irregular intervals.

As previously stated, the disease is most active before menopause, and is rare in post-menopausic women. The variations in the frequency of the disease according to age tend to support the hypothesis that it is linked to abnormal ovarian function.

FCD rarely displays symptoms until the patient discovers a palpable tumor. The tumor may be permanent, or it may appear only during the pre-menstrual phase.

Cysts which expand and contract with the menstrual cycle may be painful, as the expansion phase often develops rapidly (often contracting rapidly also, to the point where the cyst is no longer palpable).

There are numerous other cysts which must be differentiated from FCD:

-**Cysts associated with intracanicular papiloma.**

-**Cysts containing thick milky material (milk cysts)**

-**Cysts stemming from fat necrosis (oily cysts).**

-**Cysts that develop due to ductal ectasia.**

-**Pseudocysts caused by silicone injections.**

-**Sebaceous cysts.**

-**Hydatid cysts.**

-**Cysts associated with carcinomas.**

Simple Cysts

Cysts are often differentiated by size and number:

a) **According to number:**
   -Solitary or single cyst.
   -Multiple or polycystic.
b) **According to size:**
   -Microcysts, without clinical (evidence).
   -Macrocysts, which vary in size from a few milimeters to several centimeters.

A single palpable cyst will generally present itself as a hard nodule, elastic and mobile when palpated. Growth is generally slow (but if fast growth occurs, it is often painful).

Sonographically, the simple cyst has the following characteristics:
   -**Round or oval shape.**
   -**Anechoic.**
   -**Smooth and well-defined borders.**
   -**Posterior acoustic enhancement, a signal which will depend on the characterisitcs of the cyst** (size, type), **the glandular tissues, and the incidence angle of the ultrasound beam.**
   -**Lateral acoustic shadow** (which also depends upon the above mentioned parameters).

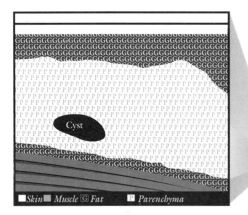

Fig. 3.1 Image of a breast with antecedent of diffuse dysplasic mastopathy which shows a cyst within a dysplasic area of 4 x 7 mm (image chromo-treated in order to outline the borders).

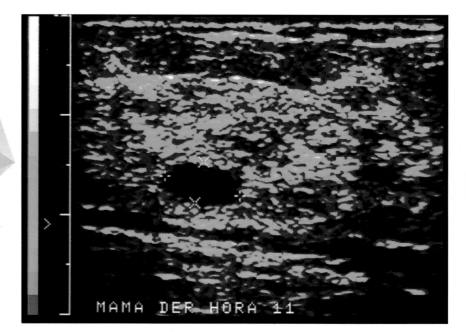

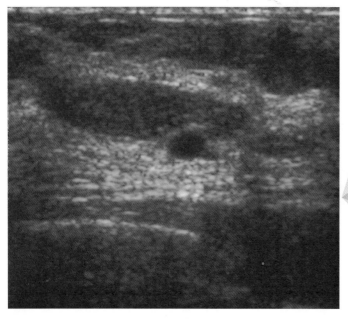

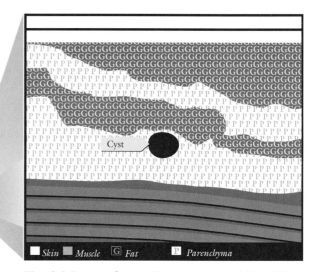

Fig. 3.2 Image of a cyst (3mm, non-palpable) within a breast with abundant fatty tissue.

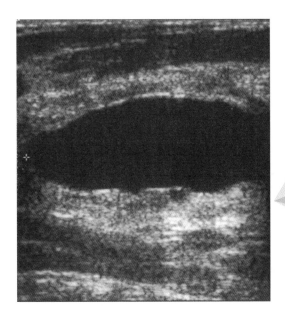

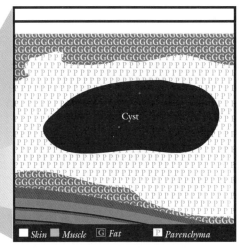

Fig. 3.3 Image of a simple cyst. Anechoic, 35mm, with smooth and regular borders and reinforcement of the posterior wall.

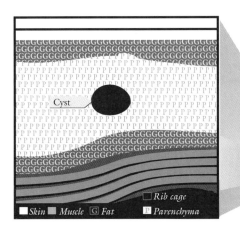

Fig. 3.4 Image of a simple cyst in a 38 year-old patient. The parenchyma is normal for the age of the patient; the cyst appears as a echonegative image 0.71mm in size.

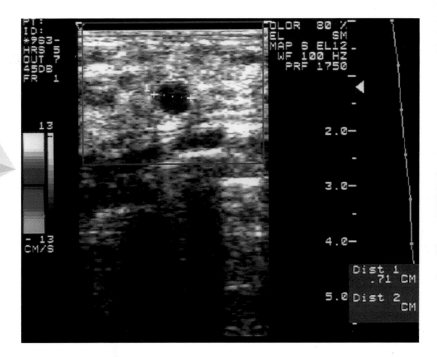

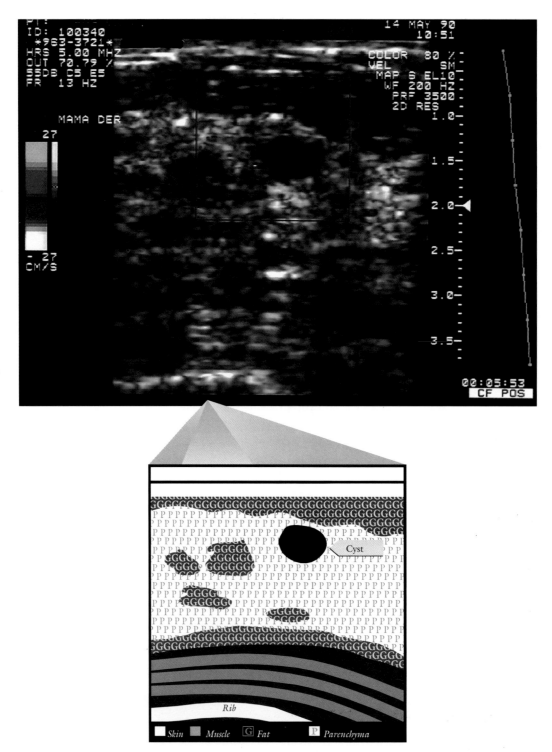

Fig. 3.5 Image of a simple cyst. Anechoic, non-palpable, 3 x 4 mm, with defined borders.

Diagnosis of a cyst by ultrasound is highly sensitive (between 98 and 100% correct). For this reason, therapeutic treatment is not normally needed, unless clinically indicated. The high reliability of ultrasound makes it a good counterpart to mammography in the task of producing well-defined images of lesions, facilitating the diferentiation between simple cysts and other pathologies such as:

-**Fibroadenoma.**
-**Solid tumor with low echogenicity** (medular, mucinous, lymphoma).
-**Lipoma.**
-**Hamartoma.**
-**Intramammary lymph node.**
-**Abscess.**
-**Galactocele.**

It must be kept in mind that cysts smaller than 3mm normally cannot be detected by ultrasound. Also, in some cases simple cysts may be bilobulated or may contain one or more fine septums.

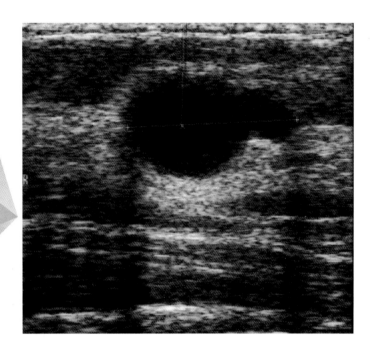

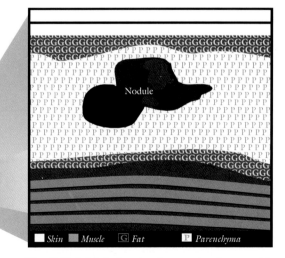

Fig. 3.6 Image of a bilobulated simple cyst. Palpable, 18 mm in size, located 11mm from the skin.

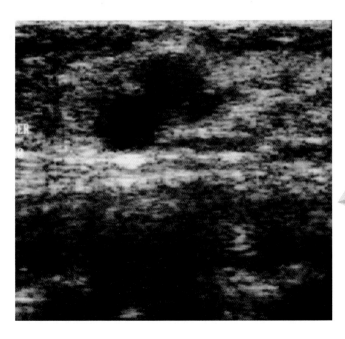

Fig. 3.7 A bilobulated echonegative image with fine interior echoes. Liquid obtained by puncture revealed an infected inflammatory process.

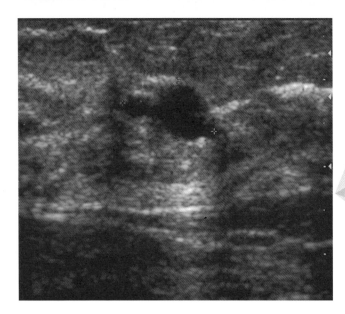

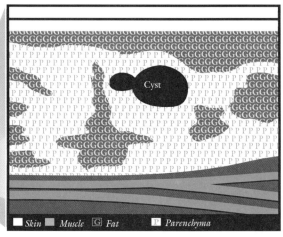

Fig. 3.8 Image of a cyst in a patient with antecedents of FCD. The cyst is a liquid-filled, bilobulated nodule which produces an anechoic ultrasound image.

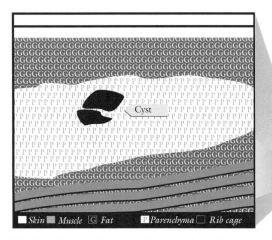

Fig. 3.9 Image of a cyst with a septum. The cyst is within the mammary parenchyma and appears as an anechoic mass with a lineal separation (image chromo-treated in order to show borders).

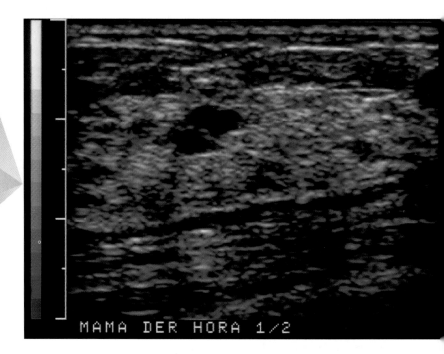

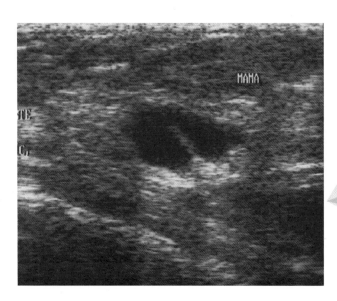

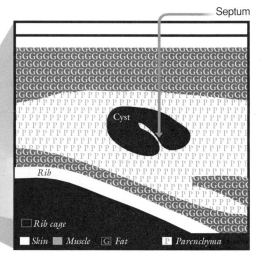

Fig. 3.10 Image of an anechoic cyst with a thin septum.

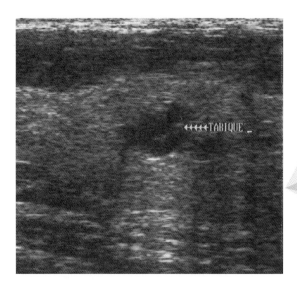

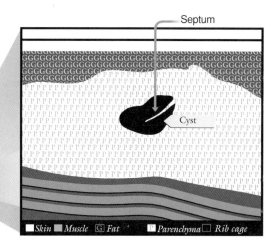

Fig. 3.11 Anechoic image of a cyst with a thin septum.

If the image of the cyst appears elongated it may be difficult to distinguish from a ductal dilation. In some cases multiple cysts may be found in one or both breasts. These cysts are usually of various sizes, and as many as 20 or 30 may be present (in such cases palpation reveals a gland which is completely irregular).

Sometimes multiple nodularity may be associated with adenosis and may include both hyperplastic and involutive lesions.

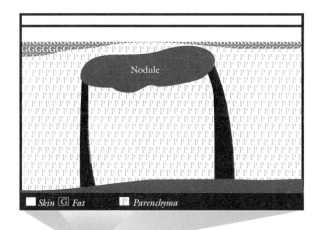

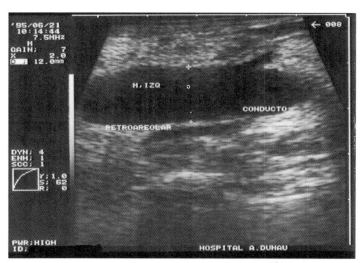

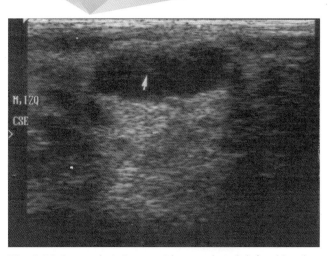

Fig. 3.12 An anechoic image with smooth and defined borders and reinforcement of the posterior wall. A lateral acoustic shadow displays small echoes in the anterior wall, due to reverberation.

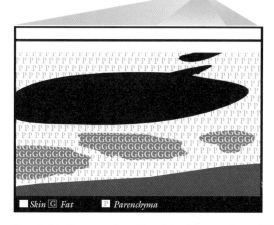

Fig. 3.13 Image of a dilated lactiferous duct. The image is anechoic, elongated, and fluid-filled, making it easy to be confused with a cystic mass.

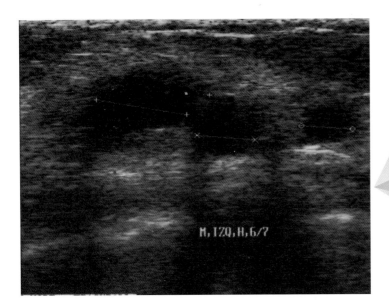

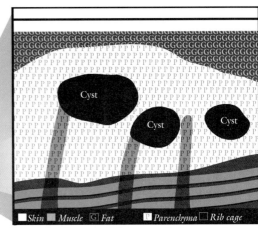

Fig. 3.14 Image of three anechoic cysts situated close to one another which display lateral sonic attenuation in a 23 year-old patient with antecedents of FCD.

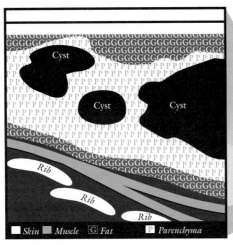

Fig. 3.15 Image of simple cysts, which appear as anechoic areas within mammary parenchyma.

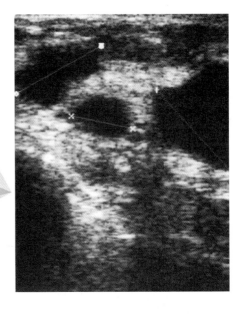

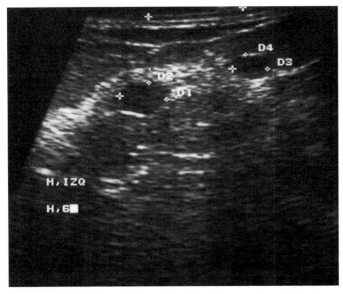

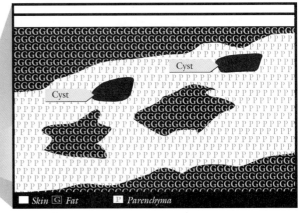

Fig. 3.16 Image of two non-palpable cysts (8 and 6mm in size) in a 40 year-old patient diagnosed with FCD and multiple cysts.

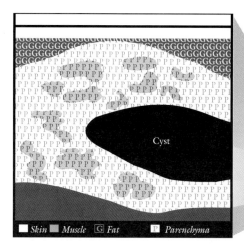

Fig. 3.17 Image of a simple cyst; bilobulated, anechoic and with defined borders within completely heterogeneous parenchyma due to FCD

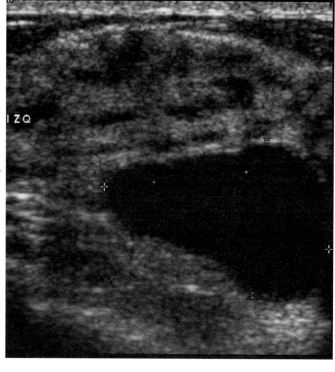

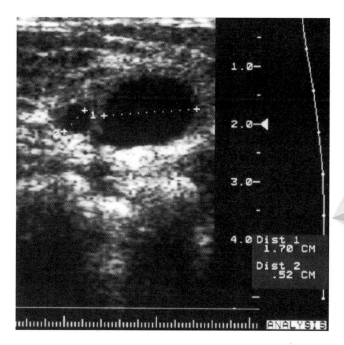

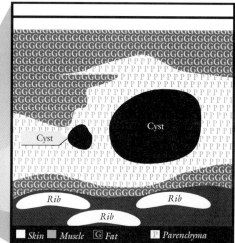

Fig. 3.18 Image of two simple cysts close to one another; anechoic, with reinforcement of the posterior wall.

Complex Cysts

Simple cysts which present complications are referred to as complex cysts. There are a number of conditions which cause complex cysts, such as:

- **Infection.**
- **Hemorrhage** (by contusion, closed trauma or post-puncture)
- **Cells in suspension.**
- **Calcifications on the cyst wall.**

Complex cysts may appear as solid images of low echogenicity, or as mixed images (both liquid and solid).

If the echoes converge on one area of the cyst wall it may be necessary to perform a differential diagnosis with an intracystic tumor. If the complex cyst contains cells in suspension due to purulent material or hemorrhage the echoes will move when the cyst is compressed or palpated.

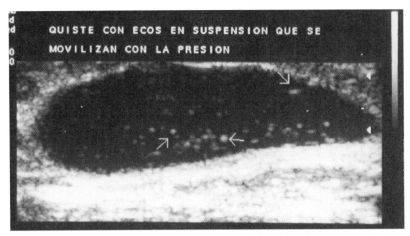

QUISTE CON ECOS EN SUSPENSION QUE SE MOVILIZAN CON LA PRESION

Fig. 3.19 Image of a cyst with smooth and defined borders; anechoic with small echoes in suspension.

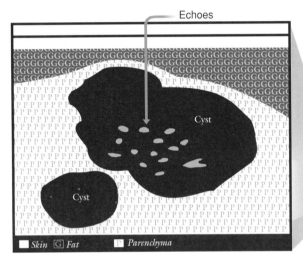

Echoes

Cyst

Cyst

☐ Skin G Fat P Parenchyma

Fig. 3.20 Image of a cyst with defined borders; anechoic, 16mm in diameter located deep within the gland. Puncture produced a greenish liquid, due to chronic galactophoritis.

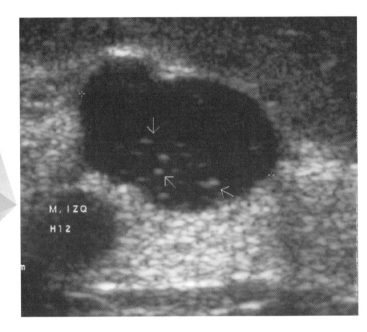

M, IZQ
H12

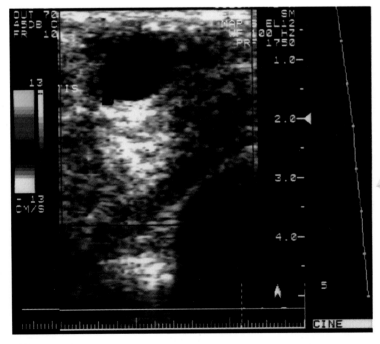

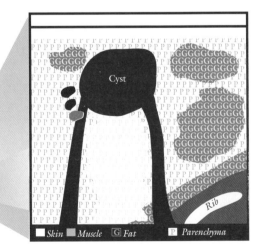

Cyst

Rib

☐ Skin ☐ Muscle G Fat P Parenchyma

Fig. 3.21 Image of a cyst with signs of infection; anechoic, with smooth and defined borders and three color focuses in one sector (vascular signal).

48

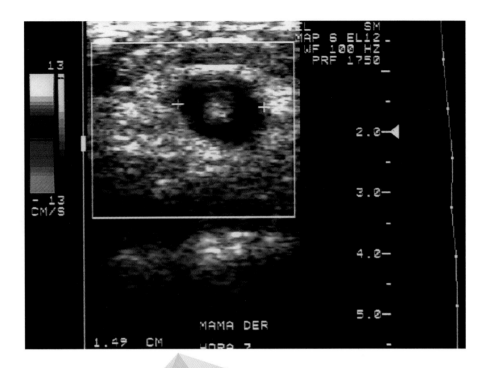

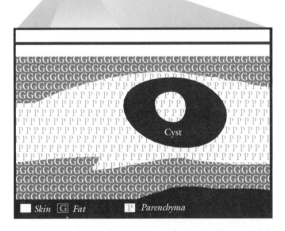

Fig. 3.22 Image of a cyst; anechoic, 1.49 cm, with defined borders and a solid mass in the center which produces an accumulation of echoes. Antecedent of cysts diagnosed by multiple punctures, which calls for a differential diagnosis.

The borders and the thin wall of a complex cyst are important because they can help differentiate cysts from necrotic tumors, intracystic tumors, or abscesses (see corresponding chapters). Occasionally, a simple cyst may take on the appearance of a complex cyst if echoes are produced by an artifact or reverberation within the superficial sector of the cyst itself. The echoes will appear as lines parallel to the skin, or as a snow effect with fine echoes within the interior of the cyst.

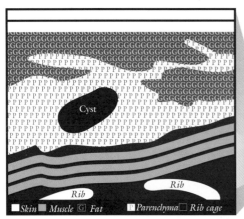

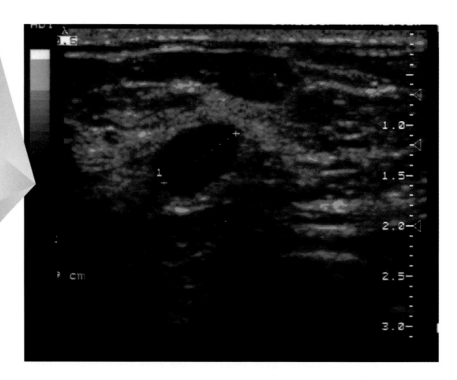

Fig. 3.23 Image of a simple cyst with slight reverberation; 0.89 cm, in a 40 year-old patient with FCD.

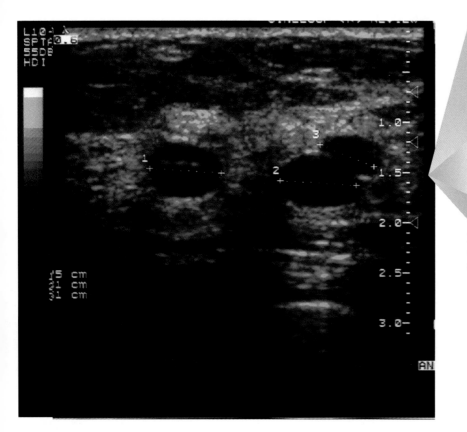

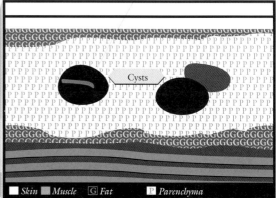

Fig. 3.24 Image of three cysts with reverberation; 0.75 cm, 0.81 cm, and 0.81 cm in size in a patient with symptoms of fibrocystic mastopathy in both breasts.

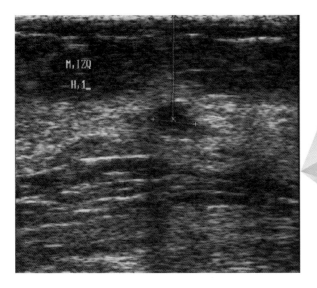

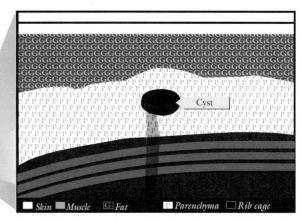

Fig. 3.25 Image of a small infected cyst with irregular borders, 6mm in size.

This effect can be counteracted by adjusting the power gain of the equipment and the angle at which the ultrasound beam strikes the lesion (ensuring that the beam bisects the lesion; see Chapter 2, "Equipment and Technique").

Cysts with pronounced fibrosis or calcified walls may produce sonic attenuation or posterior acoustic shadowing.

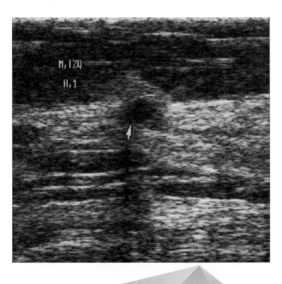

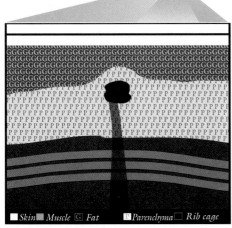

Fig. 3.26 Image of the cyst in Fig. 3.25, in which the borders appear well-defined.

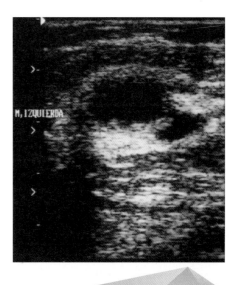

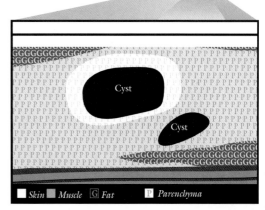

Fig. 3.27 Two anechoic images displaying thickening in the walls due to an inflammatory process.

It is difficult to produce an ultrasound image of the "calcic milk" which produces the "tea cup" signal in mammographies because of the small size of the lesions.

In some occasions the cyst wall is thickened by an inflammatory reaction in the neighboring tissues. This reaction may be the result of a puncture, or it may be spontaneous. In either case, the ultrasound image displays changes and irregularities in the borders of the cyst. Therefore, it is important to perform a differential diagnosis with an abscess.

To summarize, considering both the different forms a cyst can take and the possible complications, it is recommended that the following differential diagnoses be performed:

- **Benign or malignant intracystic tumor.**
- **Galactocele.**
- **Cyst caused by fat necrosis.**
- **Hematoma and abscess.**
- **Intratumoral necrosis.**
- **Tumors with very low echogenicity.**

When an image of a cyst displays a prolonged accumulation of echoes in one sector, there is good reason to suspect a tumor. However, the image alone is not enough to determine if it is malignant or benign.

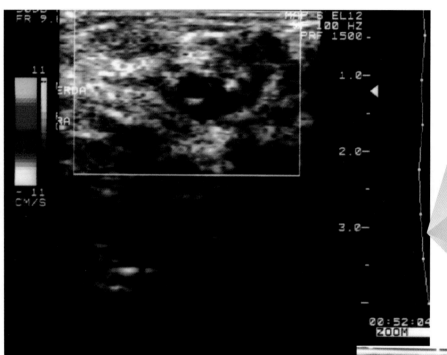

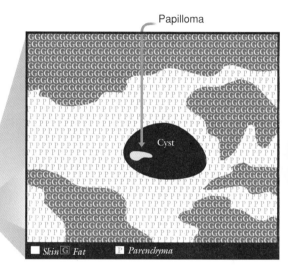

Fig. 3.28 Image of an intracystic papilloma; anechoic nodule with smooth and defined borders and echoes in one sector.

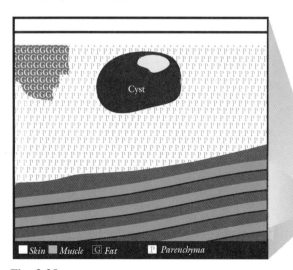

Fig. 3.29

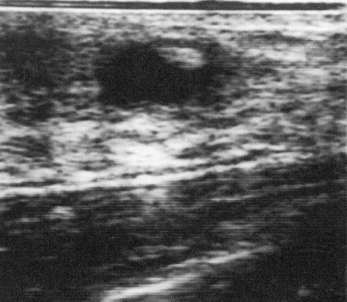

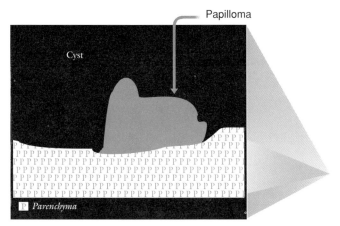

Papilloma

Cyst

P Parenchyma

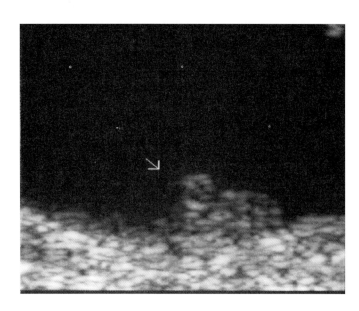

Figs. 3.30- 3.31 Images of multiple cysts which were bilateral, palpable and mobile in a 39 year-old patient. 16 simple cysts were found of various sizes between 8 and 20 mm in the right breast, and 13 simple cysts in the left breast, one of which had a vegetating image in its interior. This cyst was removed and found to be a benign papilloma.

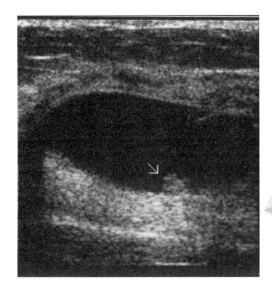

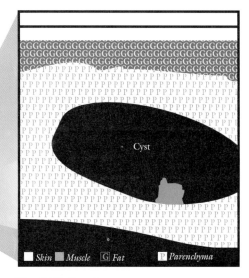

Cyst

Skin Muscle G Fat P Parenchyma

Fig. 3.31 See above.

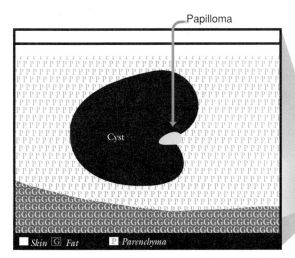

Papilloma

Cyst

Skin G Fat P Parenchyma

Fig. 3.32 Anechoic image of a palpable cyst which shows a grouping of echoes in one sector which indicates a papilloma.

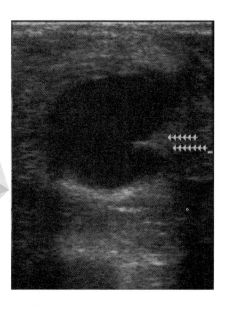

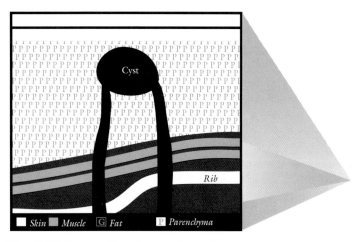
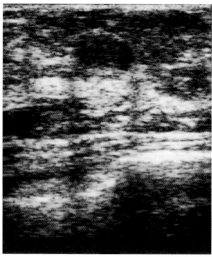

Fig. 3.33 Image of an intracystic carcinoma which appears as a hypoechoic nodule with defined borders.

Ultrasound images of galactoceles (or milk cysts) generally appear with fine interior echoes. As these echoes occupy the entire cyst, the cyst itself may appear to be solid. A diagnosis can be made rapidly by performing an aspiration and examining the fluid removed from the cyst.

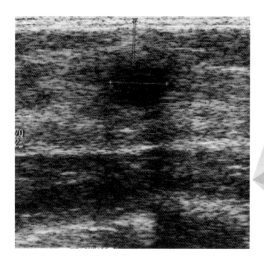
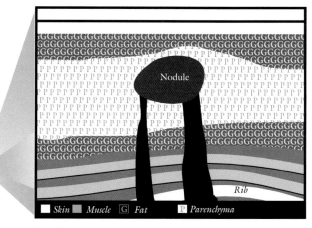

Fig. 3.34

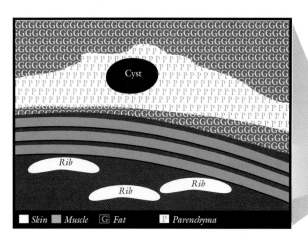
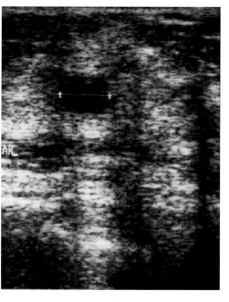

Fig. 3.35 Transverse section of a lactiferous duct, appearing as a cystic image.

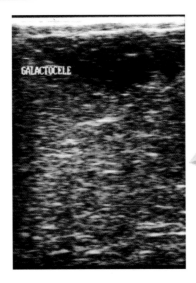

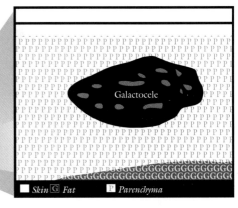

Fig. 3.36 A hypoechoic image with fine interior echoes on the superficial area of the breast which was discovered to be a galactocele.

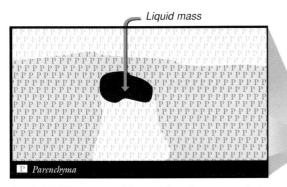

Fig. 3.37 Silicone mastitis manifested as an anechoic nodule with posterior reinforcement due to liquid content. A soft, fixed nodule was palpable close to the nipple. Patient was 34 years of age, with antecedents of a silicone injection two years previous which became infected and led to septicemia and a 3rd degree coma. A bilateral adenomammectomy was later performed.

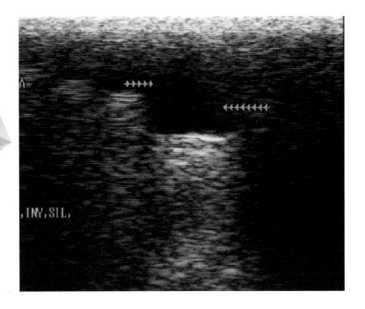

Ultrasound images of cysts caused by fat necrosis take on one of two possible appearances, either that of a simple cyst, or that of a cyst with both calcified walls (easily verified by mammography) and partial or total sonic attenuation (see Chapter 10).

Silicone injected into a breast often appears as multiple cyst-like anechoic images (although without walls). Palpation reveals exaggerated irregularity or nodulation in the entire breast, and an inmobility of these structures within the gland, as they are fixed (trapped) within the tissues.

Ultrasound-guided (US-guided) intervention is appropriate in some cases in order to aid in the diagnosis or aspiration of a cyst.

Diagnosis can be made once one has obtained a sample of fluid from the cyst. Simple cysts generally produce transparent or amber-hued samples. Reddish samples indicate the presence of red blood cells or hemorrhagic complications.

When the lesion is produced by the dilation of a lactiferous duct with a chronic inflammatory process the sample may be green or bluish. Samples taken from galactoceles tend to be milky, and purulent in cases of infection.

In cases where the lesions are painful or contain large amounts of fluid aspiration is therapeutic.

The term "ultrasound-guided (US-guided) puncture" is used in cases where the entire puncture and aspiration process is controlled with the aid of sonography.

Aspirations performed in this manner are safer and more thorough in that it is possible to ensure the successful evacuation of fluid from the cyst. In cases of cysts with septums, the procedure should be repeated in each compartment until the image disappears completely.

If an intracystic tumor is suspected this procedure should not be used. Excision is preferable in these cases, so the tissue can be subjected to anatomical-pathological study.

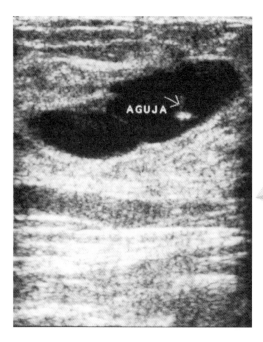

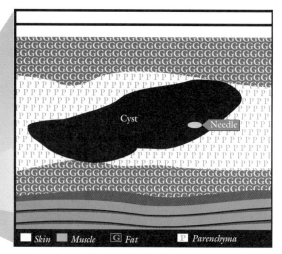

Figs. 3.38, 3.39, 3.40 Images of a galactocele (taken during the lactation period) which appears as an anechoic nodule with well-defined borders and discrete lateral sonic attenuation.

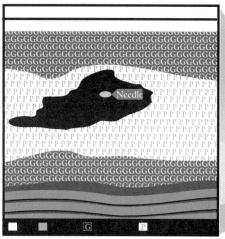

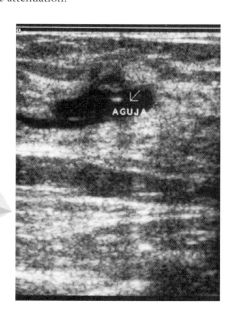

Fig. 3.39 See above.

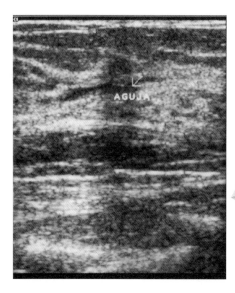

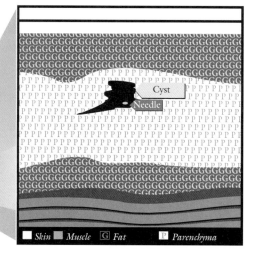

Fig. 3.40 See above.

References

- Rosen PP, Cantrell B, Muller DL, *et al.:* Juvenile papillomatosis (Swiss cheese disease) of the breast. *Am J Surg Pathol* 1980; 4:3-12.

- Rosen PP: Papillary duct hyperplasia of the breast in children and young adults. *Cancer,* 1985; 56:1611-1617.

- Kersschot EA, Hermans ME, Pauwels C *et al.:* Juvenile paillomatosis of the breast. Sonographic appearance. *Radiology* 1988; 169:631-633.

- Cole-Beuglet C, Soriano R, Kurt A *et al.:* Ultrasound, X-ray mamography and histopathology of cystocarcinoma phylloides. *Radiology,* 1983; 146:481-486.

- Mourou MY, Pujol J, Lamarque JL: La tumeur Phyllode du sein. Approche diagnostique. Bilan actuel. *J Le Sein,* 1992; 2:9-15.

- Jackson VP: The role of US in breast imaging. *Radiology,* 1990; 177:305-311.

- Adler DD: Ultrasound of benign breast conditions. *Semin Ultrasound CT MR,* 1989; 10:106-118.

- Moskowitz M: Circunscribed lesions of the breast. In: Moskowitz M, ed.: *Syllabus: a diagnostic categorical course in breast imaging.* Oak Brook, III Radiological Society of North America, 1986; 31-33.

- Jokich PM, Monticciolo DL, Adler YT: Breast ultrasonography. *Radiol Clin North Am,* 1992; 30:993-1009.

- Jakson VP, Rothschild PA, Kreipe DL *et al.:* The spectrun of sonographic findings of fibroadenoma of the breast. *Invest Radiol,* 1986; 21:34-40.

- Cole-Beuglet C, Soriano RZ, Kurtz AB, Goldberg BB: Fibroadenoma of the brreast: sonomammography correlated with pathology in 122 patients. *AJR,* 1983; 140:369-375.

- Bassett LW, Ysrael M, Gold RH, Ysrael C: Usefulness of mammography and sonography in women les than 35 years old. *Radiology* 1991; 180:831-835.

- Hilton SW, Leopolod GR, Olson LK, Wilson SA: Real-time breastsonography application in 300 consecutive patients. *AJR,* 1986; 147:479-486.

- Vlaisavljevic: Differentation of solid breast tumors on the basis of their primary echographic characteristics as revealed by real-time scanning of the uncompressed breast. *Ultrasound Med Biol,* 1988; 14 (suppl 1):59-73.

- Hackeloer B-J, Duda V, Lauth G: *Ultrasound Mammography.* Springer-Verlag, New York, 1989.

- Jackson VP, Rothschild PA, Kreipke DL *et al.:* The spectrum sonographic findings of fibroadenoma of the breast. *Invest Radiol,* 1986; 34-40.

- Formage BD, Lorigan JG, Andry E: Fibroadenoma of the breast: sonographic appearane. *Radiology,* 1989; 172:671-675.

- Cole-Beuglet C, Soriano RZ, Kurtz, AB, Goldberg, BB: Fibroadenoma of the breast: sonomammography correlated with pathology in 122 patients. *AJR,* 1983; 140:369-375.

- Moran CS: Fibroadenoma of the breast during pregnancy and lactation. *Arch Surg,* 1935; 31:688-708.

- Kopans DB, Meyer JE, Proppe KH: Ultrasonographic, xeromammographic and histologic correlation of a fibroadenolipoma of the breast. *J Clin Ultrasound,* 1982; 10:409-411.

- Adler DD, Jeffries DO, Helvie MA: Sonographic features of breast hamartomas. *J Ultrasound Med,* 1990; 9:85-90.

- Spalding JE: Adeno-lipoma and lipoma of the breast. *Guy's Hosp Rep,* 1945; 94: 80-84.

- Strickles EA, Filly RA, Callen PW: Benign breast lesions: ultrasound detection and diagnosis. *Radiology,* 151: 1984; 467-470.

- Byrd BF, Hartmann, WH, Graham LS, Hogle HH: Mastopathy in insulin-dependent diabeties. *Ann Surg,* 205: 1987; 529-532.

- Gartstin WIH, Aufmann ZK, Michell MJ, Baum M: Fibrous mastopathy in insulin dependent diabetes. *Clin Radio* 1991, 44: 89-91.

Solid Benign Nodule

M. E. Lanfranchi

Benign solid nodules are a common pathology. They can be divided into six basic types:

- **Fibroadenoma.**
- **Phyllodes tumor.**

- **Focal dysplasic papillomatosis.**
- **Nipple adenoma.**
- **Benign soft tissue tumors of the breast.**
- **Benign skin tumors of the breast.**

Fibroadenoma

Fibroadenoma affects young women, primarily those between 15 and 35 years of age. Nodules found in older patients usually develop in this time period, but go undetected for years. These nodules are mobile, well-circumscribed, and have a firm, elastic consistency. They do not retract or adhere to the skin.

They are usually painless and grow rather slowly, developing in several months or even years (especially those in which connective tissue is predominant).

Fibroadenoma is a relatively common pathology which develops in otherwise healthy parenchyma. It manifests itself as a solid, well-defined oval or round nodule, which may display a number of lobulations. Fibroadenomas are composed of epithelial and connective tissue, and their echostructure is generally homogeneous. They may be bilateral (9.9%) and/or multiple (10% to 16% of cases).

According to a hospital study conducted by J.V. Uriburu, 3.5 fibroadenomas are found for every 1 carcinoma.

In ultrasound images fibroadenomas generally display an increase in the number of echoes in the posterior wall, and a faint lateral sonic attenuation.

Nodule size is variable, usually reaching a maximum of 2 to 2.5 cm, although in cases of giant juvenile fibroadenoma maximum size may reach 8 to 10 cm.

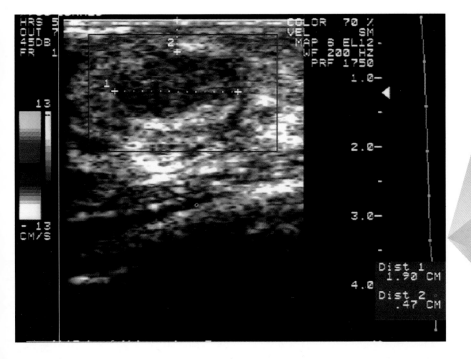

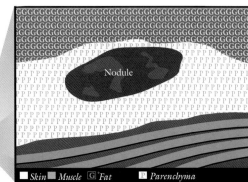

Fig. 4.1 Image of a solid mass with well-defined borders and large lobulations in a 19 year-old patient who complained of a palpable nodule. The mass was diagnosed as a fibroadenoma.

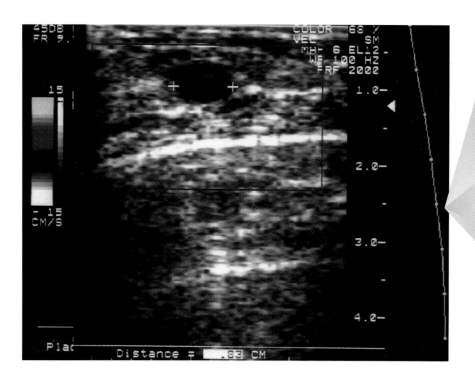

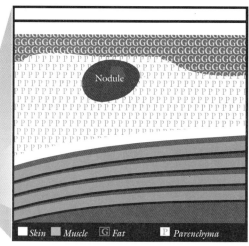

Fig. 4.2 Image of a solid mass, 8mm in diameter displaying low echogenicity and smooth and defined borders. The mass was diagnosed as a nodular dysplasia with adenosis.

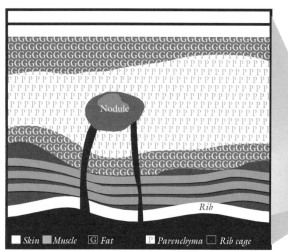

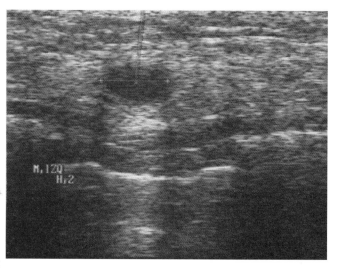

Fig. 4.3 Image of a homogeneous non-palpable nodule 7mm in diameter and located at a depth of 10 mm. The nodule displayed regular borders and discrete lateral sonic attenuation and was diagnosed as an adenolipoma.

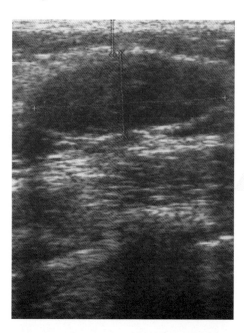

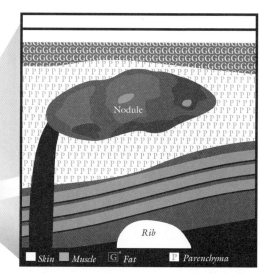

Fig. 4.4 Image of a relatively homogeneous solid nodule with well-defined borders in a 39 year-old patient. It was diagnosed as a fibroadenoma.

When a young woman experiences considerable augmentation in one of the breasts, there are three pathologies which should be considered:
- **Giant fibroadenoma.**
- **Unilateral virginal hypertrophy.**
- **Phyllodes tumor.**

Giant fibroadenoma, as its name implies, is a large, palpable, circumscribed nodule. It has all the characteristics of a benign nodule, and does not infiltrate the surrounding tissue.

Virginal hypertrophy is diffuse; there is an augmentation of the entire gland, but no definite nodule formation.

The phyllodes tumor is a large, somewhat heterogeneous, circumscribed nodule, which may have lobulations.

Differential diagnosis to determine nodule type is only possible by a postsurgical histological study.

There may be alterations in some fibroadenomas, calcification being the most frequent.

Focal calcifications appear as areas of high echogenicity in one sector of the nodule, either with or without posterior attenuation.

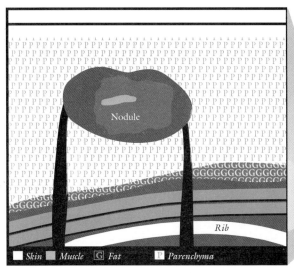

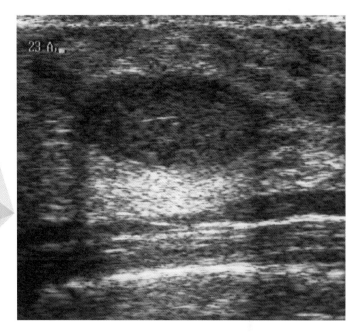

Fig. 4.5 Image of a solid nodule with regular and well-defined borders in a 23 year-old patient who complained of a mobile palpable nodule. The nodule was diagnosed as a fibroadenoma.

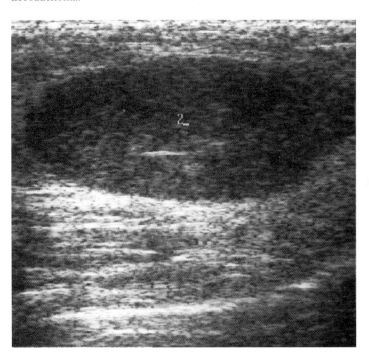

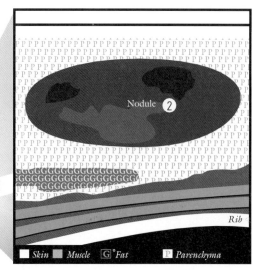

Figs. 4.6, 4.7, 4.8 Images of a pair of nodules in close proximity which resembled a single nodule during physical examination. Both nodules had regular and well-defined borders and produced homogeneous echoes. The nodules were diagnosed as fibroadenomas.

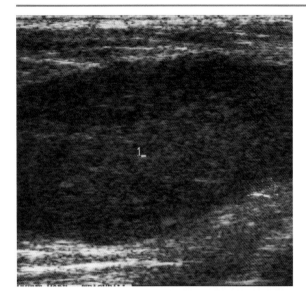

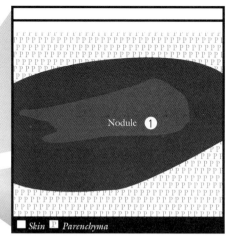

Fig. 4.7 See above.

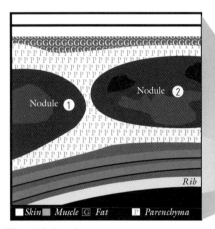

Fig. 4.8 See above.

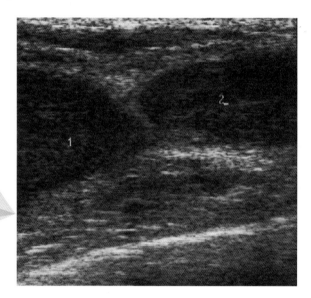

When the fibroadenoma is heavily calcified, or calcifications are located in the superficial sector of the nodule, the image generally appears completely heterogeneous, with partial or total sonic attenuation.

In cases of complete posterior acoustic shadowing, the image is indistinguishable from that of some cancers.

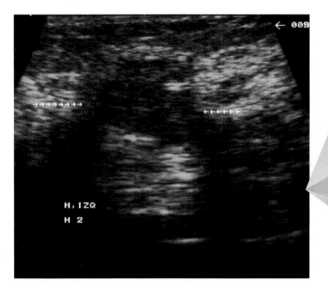

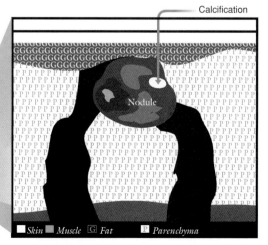

Fig. 4.9 Image of a solid nodule with large lobulations and interior calcifications which produced lateral sonic attenuation. The nodule was diagnosed as a fibroadenoma.

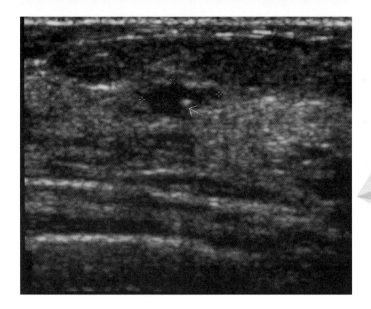

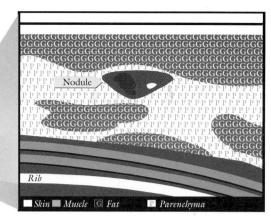

Fig. 4.10 Image of a non-palpable nodule 7mm in diameter with defined borders and a single lobulation which also displayed calcifications. It was diagnosed as a fibroadenoma.

In such cases it is wise to combine mammographical and ultrasound studies in order to facilitate diagnosis.

In cases of hemorrhage or necrosis within the fibroadenoma, the ultrasound image of the nodule will

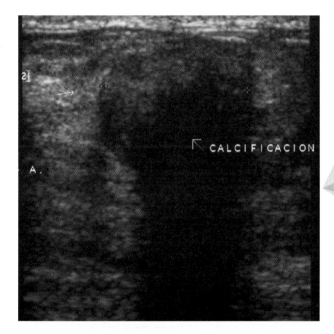

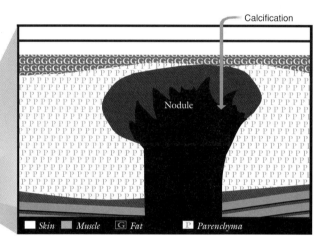

Figs. 4.11- 4.15 Images of a solid nodule with well-defined borders in its anterior portion and considerable sonic attenuation in its lower portion in a 24 year-old patient who complained of a palpable nodule. As figures 4.12-4.15 indicate, another nodule with similar characteristics was found in close proximity with this nodule.

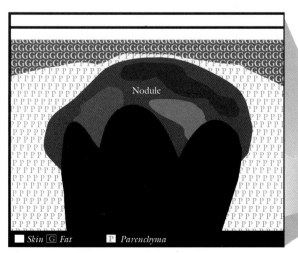

Fig. 4.12 See above.

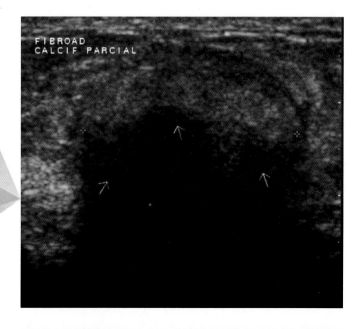

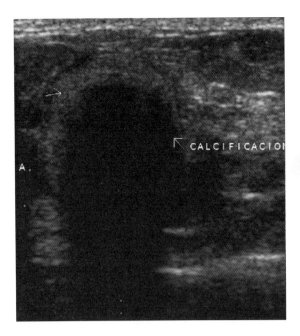

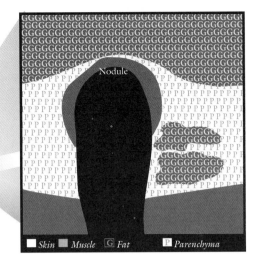

Fig. 4.13 See above.

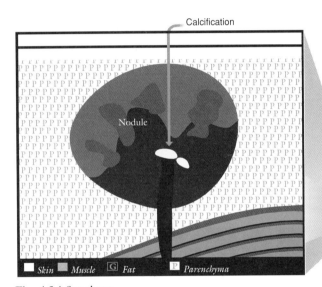

Fig. 4.14 See above.

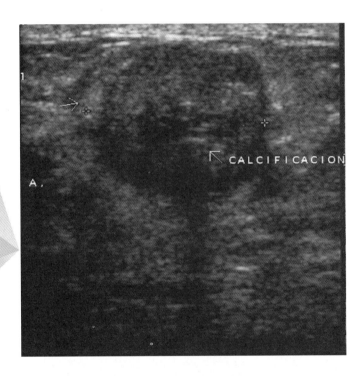

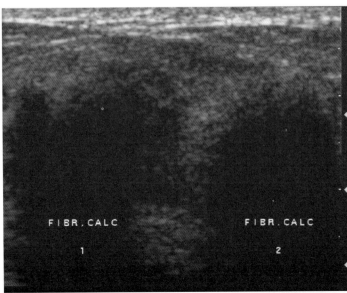

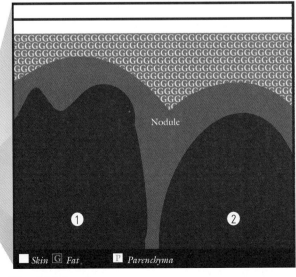

Fig. 4.15 See above.

generally be completely heterogeneous, with both solid and liquid areas. Both hemorrhage and necrosis can cause a rapid increase in the volume of the nodule, forcing one to differenciate it from a cancer.

Numerous variations are possible in the ultrasound images of fibroadenomas. The five most common are listed below:

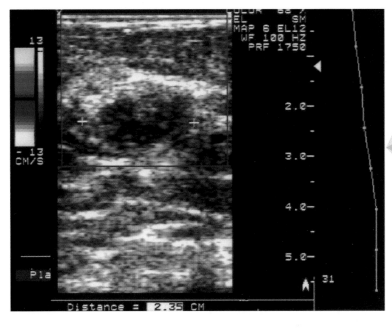

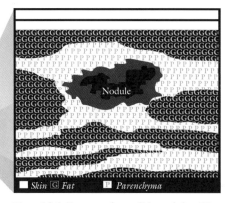

Fig. 4.16 Image of a solid nodule, 20 x 14mm in size, with defined borders in a patient with an antecedent of a burn on the left breast. The echostructure of the nodule was heterogeneous due to a transformation of the interior tissues which. The nodule was diagnosed as a fibroadenoma.

Variations in the Appearance of Fibroadenomas

1) **Elongated shape, with smooth borders and heterogeneous echostructure.**

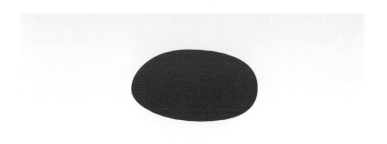

Figure 4.17

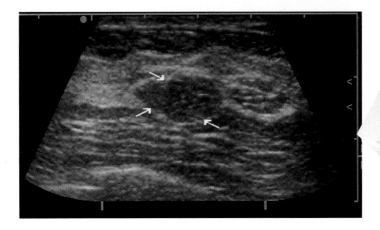

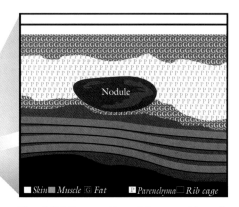

Fig. 4.18 Image of a solid mass with well-defined borders. The mass was diagnosed as a fibroadenoma.

2) Bilobular or trilobular shape.

a

Figure 4.19

b

Figure 4.20

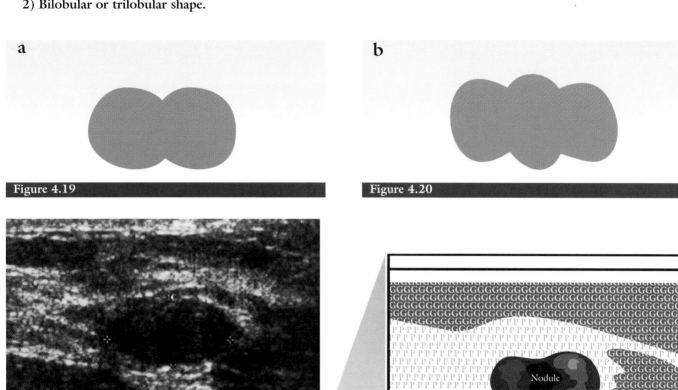

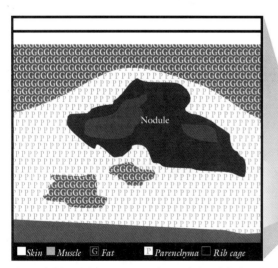

Fig. 4.21 Image of a solid bilobulated nodule with regular, defined borders. The nodule was diagnosed as a fibroadenoma.

Skin ▪ Muscle G Fat P Parenchyma

Skin ▪ Muscle G Fat P Parenchyma ▫ Rib cage

Figs. 4.22, 4.23 Images of a solid trilobulated nodule with sharp borders which seems to present sonic attenuation in one sector. The nodule was diagnosed as a fibroadenoma.

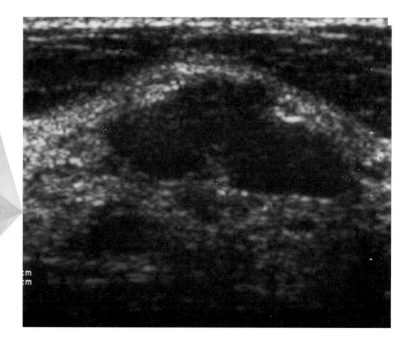

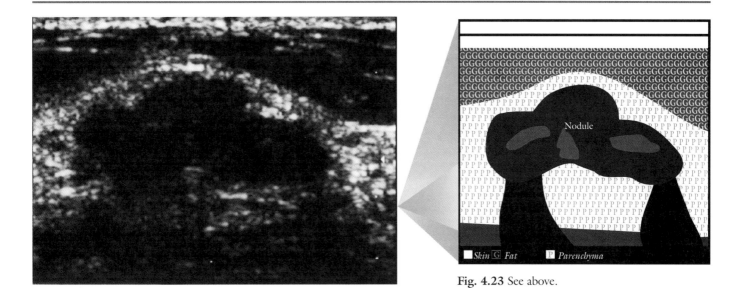

Fig. 4.23 See above.

3) Containing a small area of partial calcification; with or without posterior sonic attenuation.

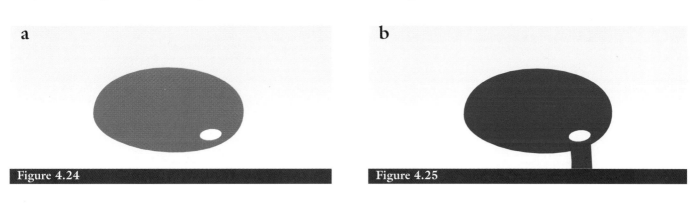

Figure 4.24

Figure 4.25

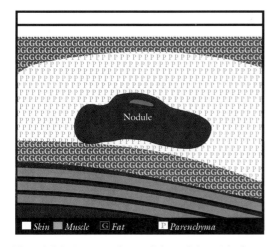

Fig. 4.26 Image of a solid nodule with large lobulations and an area of greater echogenicity in the right breast. This patient had a prior resection of a fibroadenoma in the same breast. Histological diagnosis: fibroadenoma.

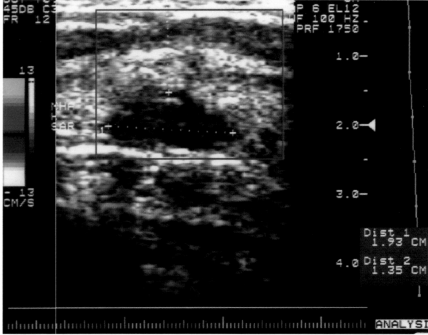

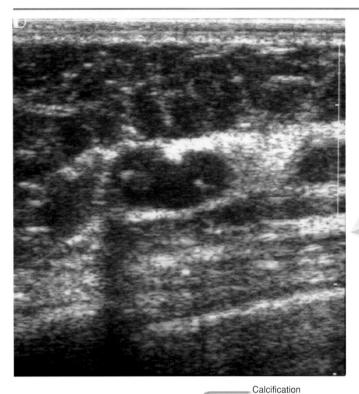

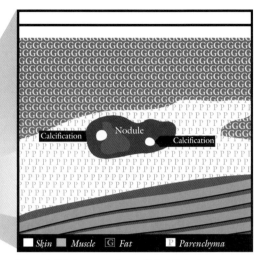

Fig. 4.27 Image of a solid, bilobulated, non-palpable nodule with defined borders found within a dysplasic mass. Fibroadenoma.

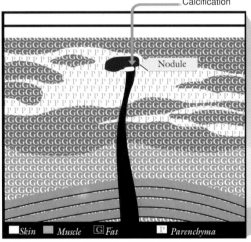

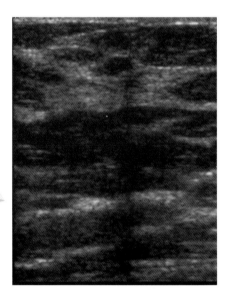

Fig. 4.28 Image of a non-palpable nodule, 5mm in size which contains a calcification on one border. Fibroadenoma.

4) Displaying thick calcifications and total sonic attenuation.

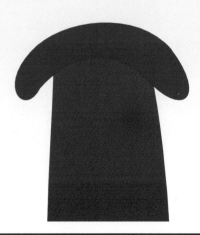

Figure 4.29

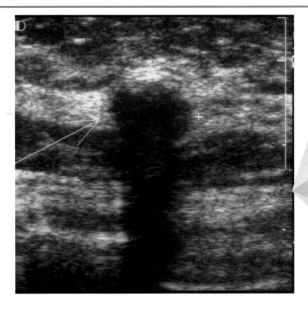

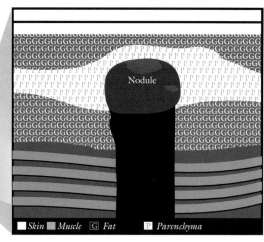

Fig. 4.30 Image of a solid nodule, 11mm in size, in a patient who had been diagnosed with a calcified fibroadenoma by mammography. In this image only the anterior portion can be seen due to strong sonic attenuation caused by the calcification.

5) Heterogeneous, with hemorrhage and/or necrosis.

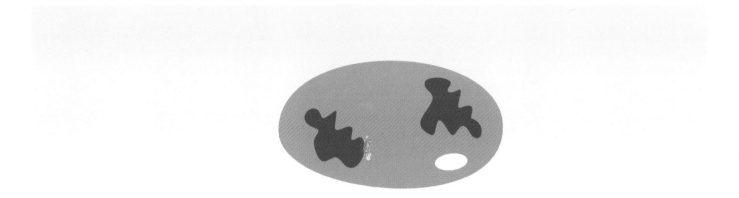

Figure 4.31

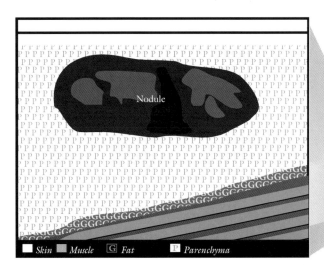

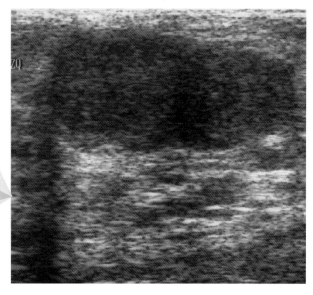

Fig. 4.32 Image of a solid, relatively heterogeneous nodule with defined borders. Fibroadenoma.

Fibroadenoma rarely becomes malignant. However, due to its composition it may transform into a carcinoma or sarcoma with a low degree of malignancy.

Carcinomas within fibroadenomas are also quite rare (0.3%, according Ozello). Haagensen found only two cases of lobular carcinoma *in situ* within a fibroadenoma, both of which were cured by resection. In a study published in 1989 Dent and Cant stated that, globally, there were only ninety-six cases of cancers within fibroadenomas.

Nonetheless, the author herself encountered a case of a tumor measuring 1cm which, when examined using Doppler color, revealed itself to be a fibroadenoma with a carcinoma in one sector.

It is worth noting that carcinomas may appear in the same breast along with a fibroadenoma, or in the contralateral breast. Carcinomas may also present themselves in patients who have undergone surgery for fibroadenoma.

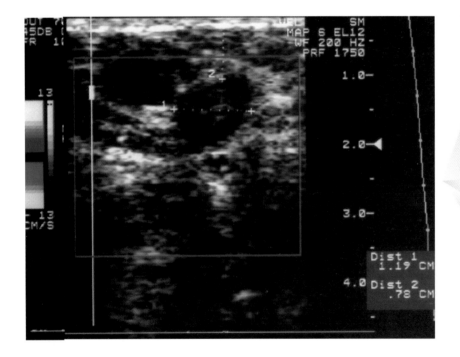

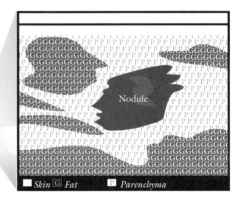

Fig. 4.33 Image of a solid hypoechoic nodule 11 x 7mm in diameter with sharp borders and an irregularity in two sectors. It was diagnosed as a fibroadenoma with an eccentric carcinomatous concentration.

Differential Diagnosis of Fibroadenoma

In the differential diagnosis of fibroadenomas other circumscribed nodules with a similar ultrasound appearance must be included:

- **Phyllodes tumor** (see corresponding section).
- **Zone of adenosis**
- **Fibrocystic disease.**

- **Certain carcinomas** (such as medullary and mucinous carcinomas).
- **Papillary tumors** (in retroareolar or juxtaareolar locations, and often accompanied by nipple secretions.
- **Lipoma** (not as mobile; radiolucent in the mammography).

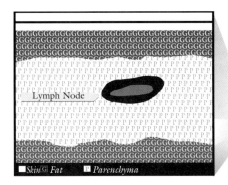

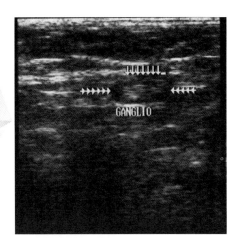

Fig. 4.34 Image of a nodule located in the middle of the parenchyma which displays a central area of greater echogenicity. It was found to be an intramammary lymph node.

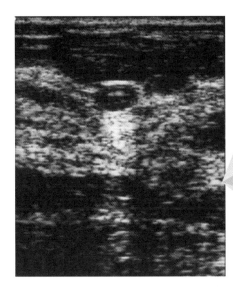

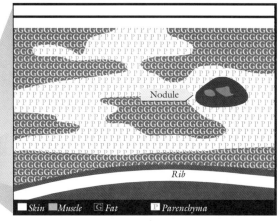

Fig. 4.35 Image of a small, solid hypoechoic nodule with a central area of greater echogenicity. Needle biopsy showed an intramammary lymph node.

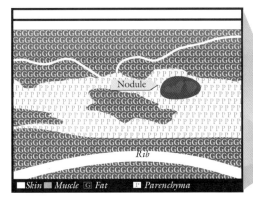

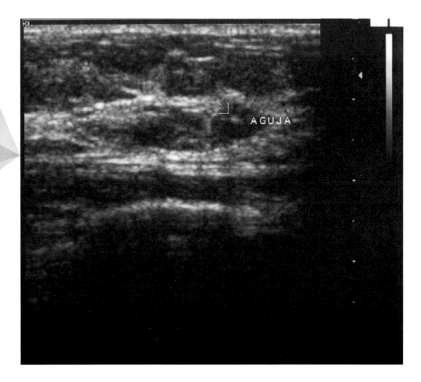

Fig. 4.36 Image of a solid, non-palpable intramammary nodule displaying low echogenicity and defined borders. The tip of the needle used for puncture can be seen. The nodule was diagnosed as a intramammary lymph node.

-**Fat necrosis** (there is a history of prior trauma).
-**Intramammary lymph node.**

Fibroadenoma is the most frequent of the benign pathologies, as Table 4.1 shows.

Pathology	Rate
Fibroadenoma	50%
Fibrosclerosis	15%
Papillary duct hyperplasia	3%
Adenosis	3%
Fibrocystic mastopathy	15%
Intraductal papilloma	2%
Others	12%
Table 4.1	

Phyllodes Tumor

The phyllodes tumor (cystosarcoma phyllodes) is a relatively rare pathology, representing 0.5 to 1% of all breast tumors, and 1 to 2% of fibroepithelial tumors of the breast.

The nature of this tumor is controversial because it has both benign and malignant variants. For example, there are documented cases of phyllodes tumors type I on the Norris and Taylor scale which degenerated into sarcomas, causing the death of the patient. On the other hand, tumors type IV on the Norris and Taylor scale have been sucessfully treated by resections.

Histologically, the phyllodes tumor can be defined as a fibroepithelial tumor which transforms into a sarcoma in 10.25% of the documented cases, and has a 15 to 20% chance of local recurrence.

The phyllodes tumor has been given many names, but currently it is known as either "phyllodes tumor" or "periductal stromal tumor". The term "pyllodes" refers to the leaf-shaped appearance of the tumor.

Phyllodes tumor may appear in the same breast as a fibroadenoma and it is possible for both pathologies to exist in the same nodule.

There have been cases of phyllodes tumor in men; according to a study by Barboza de Castro y Ribeiro, there is approximately one male case for every 100 cases in women.

Size is variable, and depends upon the stage of development at the time of discovery.

Table 4.2 below shows tumor sizes and their frequency of occurrence.

Size	%
More than 20 cm	15%
From 10 to 20 cm	36%
From 5 to 10 cm	34%
Less than 4 cm	15%
Table 4.2	

Ultrasound images of phyllodes tumors may display the following characteristics:

- **Well-defined borders.**
- **Lobulations.**
- **Areas of fibrosis.**
- **Areas of myxomatosis.**
- **Cavities filled with hemorrhagic or necrotic liquid.**

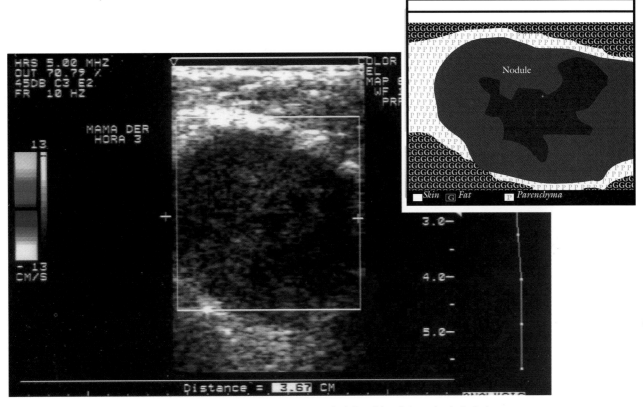

Fig. 4.37 Image of a solid, palpable nodule 36 x 39mm in size with defined borders and relatively heterogeneous echoes. Biopsy showed a phyllodes tumor.

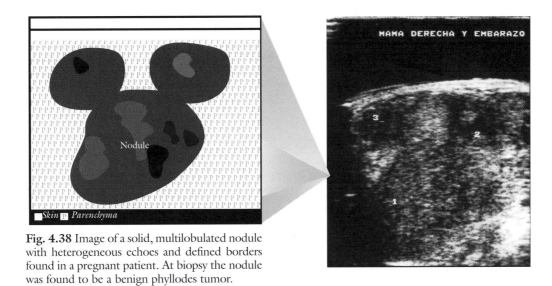

Fig. 4.38 Image of a solid, multilobulated nodule with heterogeneous echoes and defined borders found in a pregnant patient. At biopsy the nodule was found to be a benign phyllodes tumor.

73

Parenchyma adjacent to phyllodes tumors may have a laminate appearance due to displacement or compression by the tumor itself. Also, the skin overlying the tumor may be affected with cianosis or collateral venous circulation.

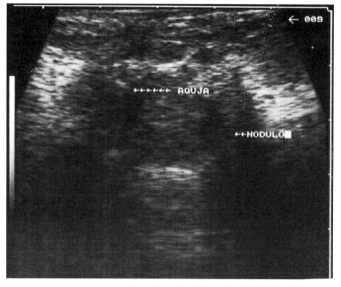
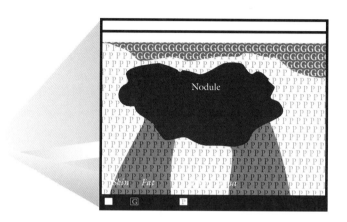

Fig. 4.39 Image of a solid, lobulated mass with areas of sonic attenuation in a patient who had undergone antecedent surgery for a phyllodes tumor. Recurrence confirmed by biopsy.

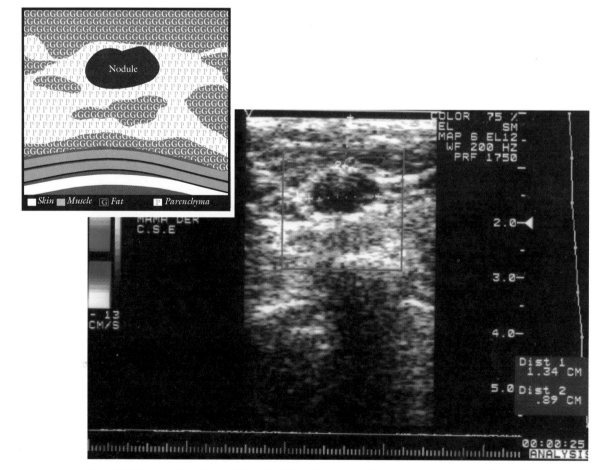

Fig. 4.40 Image of a solid nodule with defined borders and benign characteristics. It was diagnosed as a benign phyllodes tumor.

Papillomatosis

Papillomatosis is a rare non-cyclic dysplasia which typically displays a focal lesion with multiple dysplasic papillary formations.

It may display the following symptoms:

- **Discharge from the nipple.**
- **A small nodule at any point in the gland.**

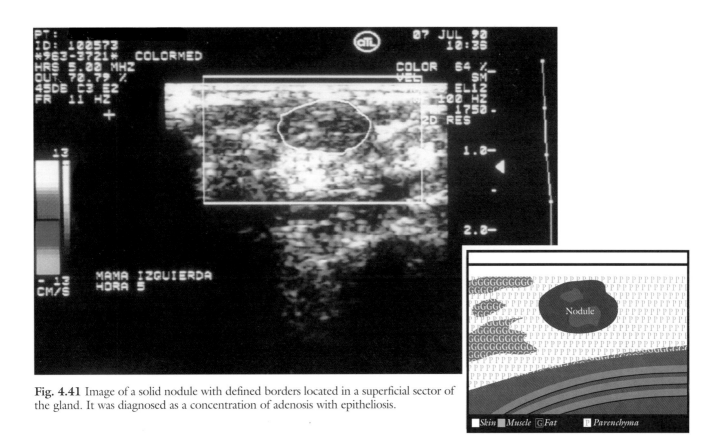

Fig. 4.41 Image of a solid nodule with defined borders located in a superficial sector of the gland. It was diagnosed as a concentration of adenosis with epitheliosis.

Nipple Adenoma

Nipple adenoma is quite rare, occurring in one of every 4,000 mastopathies, according to a study published by Gross. It normally affects the distal portion of a lactiferous duct, and manifests itself as a well-defined solid nodule a few millimeters in diameter in the area of the nipple. It may cause the nipple to appear ulcerated or scaly, and can be mistaken for Paget's disease of the breast.

Benign Soft Tissue Tumors of the Breast

There are a number of tumors which affect the breast, but are not specific to it. Geschickter divides them according to their origin:

a) Mesodermic:
- Adipose tissue: lipoma, xanthoma, fat necrosis.
- Vessels: angioma, lymphangioma.
- Muscles: leiomyoma, myoblastoma.
- Bones: chondroma, osteoma.

b) Epithelial tissue:
- Tumoral cysts of the sweat glands.

Lipomas are the most frequent benign tumors, constituting 87% of benign mammary diseases appearing in women over forty.

They may be located in the premammary or retromammary layer, or in the interior of the gland. Lipomas located in tha axilla may be mistaken for lymph nodes.

Lipomas have even borders and tend to be smooth, soft, and mobile. Their echostructure is similar to that of the subcutaneous tissues, therefore they may be difficult to detect by ultrasound.

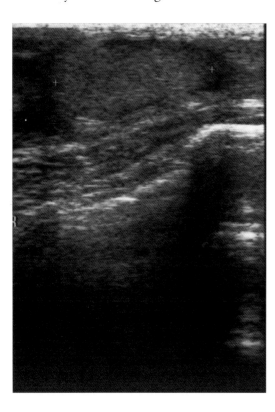

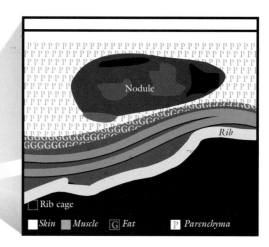

Fig. 4.42 Image of a solid nodule 22 x 11mm in size with defined borders and a predominant hyperechoic pattern. A biopsy was performed and the nodule was found to be a fibroadenolipoma.

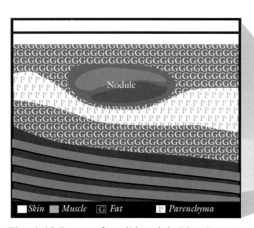

Fig. 4.43 Image of a solid nodule 12 x 8mm in size with a central area of greater echogenicity in a patient who complained of a soft, palpable nodule. Lipoma.

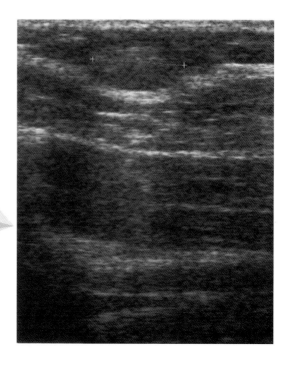

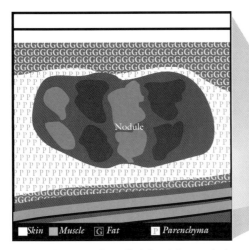
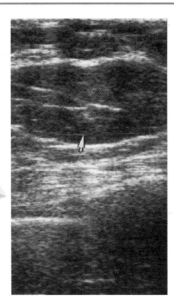

Fig. 4.44 Image of a well-defined, hypoechoic nodule which was both palpable and elastic. Lipoma.

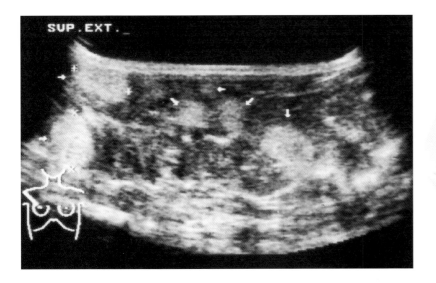

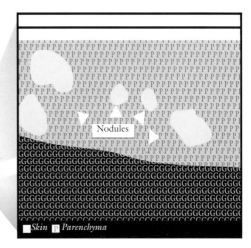

Figs. 4.45-4.47 Images of multiple small, highly echogenic nodules located in different sectors of the breast of a 71 year-old patient. Lipomas. (Images by Dr. Miguel Ariel)

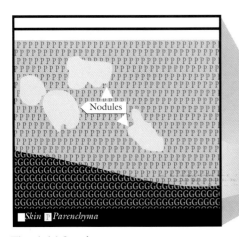

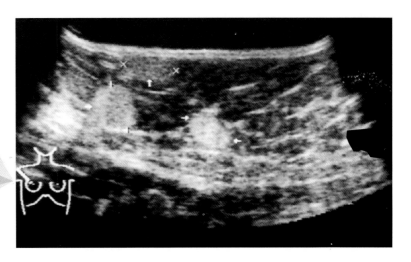

Fig. 4.46 See above.

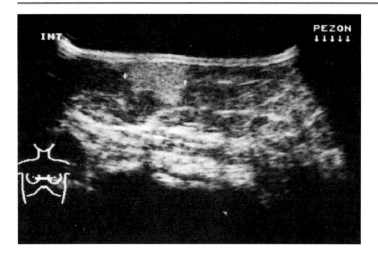

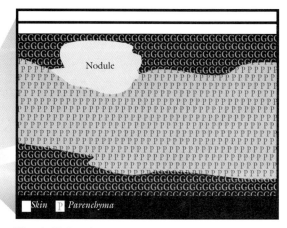

Fig. 4.47 See above.

In ultrasound images, lipomas may have an appearance similar to that of fibroadenomas. However, the former are more easily compressed during palpation.

Adenolipoma is a rare type of lipoma. Studies by investigators such as Riveros et al. and Hughes et al. suggest that it may be a type of hamartoma.

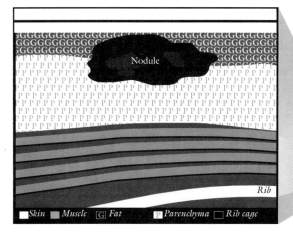

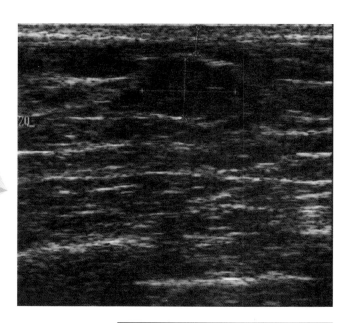

Fig. 4.48 Image of a solid nodule displaying low echogenicity and defined borders in a 55 year-old male. Fibrolipoma diagnosed by biopsy.

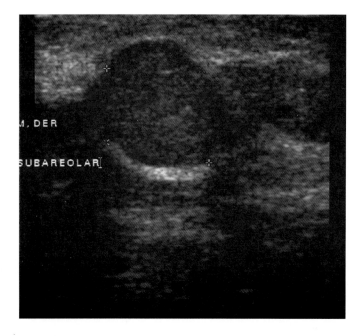

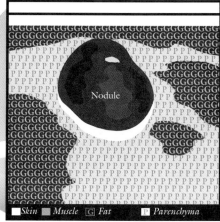

Fig. 4.49 Image of a solid, hypoechoic nodule in the subareolar region, 13 x 15mm in size, with well-defined borders. A needle biopsy confirmed it to be a fibrolipoma.

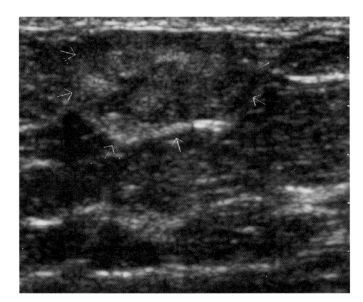

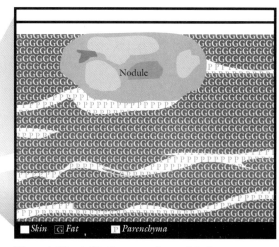

Figs. 4.50, 4.51 Images of a solid, heterogeneous nodule with areas of varying echogenicity. Diagnosed by biopsy as a fibroadenolipoma.

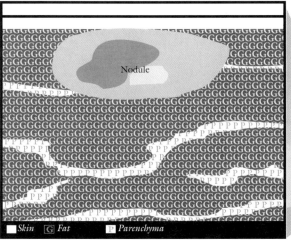

Fig. 4.51 See above.

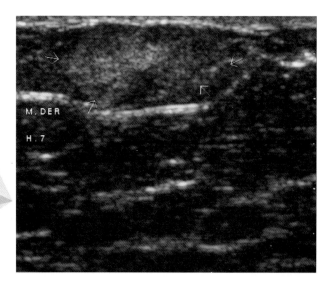

Neurofibromatosis, or Von Recklinghausen's disease can manifest itself as multiple nodules within the premammary fat. The disease can be suspected when nodules and light brown spots on the skin are found in other parts of the body.

Hamartoma, also known as adenolipoma, or chondrolipoma, is a rare, slow-growing, benign tumor which normally has an oval shape. It is mobile, does not adhere to surrounding tissues, and most often appears in women in their forties or fifties. The ultrasound image should be differentiated from those of lipoma, fibroadenoma, and phyllodes tumors.

Other rare benign tumors:

- **Benign fibrous histocytoma**: often lies just below the skin, appearing to infiltrate it. It generally manifests itself as small, well-circumscribed nodules.

- **Granular cell tumor**: easily mistaken clinically and sonographically for a carcinoma. These tumors, although benign, tend to adhere to the skin and the pectoral muscles.

- **Benign angioma**: very rare. Melville could find only seven cases of occurrence within the breast. These tend to be cavernous, non-encapsulated tumors which tend to shrink in size when compressed and are generally located within the superficial fascia.

Tumors affecting the epithelial tissue are generally tumors of the sweat glands, located under the areola or its borders. They tend to have a cystic structure and fine echoes in their interior.

Sebaceous cysts of the breast are relatively common, especially in the region of the areola. They generally occur when a hair follicle is dilated and a comedo (which may become infected and filled with pus) is formed in the skin or the subcutaneous tissue. Ultrasound images of these cysts appear on the following pages.

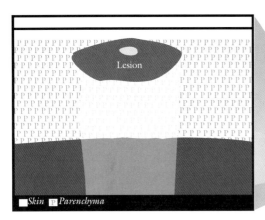

Fig. 4.52 Image of a solid nodule displaying low echogenicity, defined borders, and an area of greater heterogeneity which reaches a depth of 6mm in a patient complaining of an indurated lesion on the skin of the breast. The lesion showed signs of chronic inflammation and was diagnosed as a chronic granuloma caused by a foreign body.

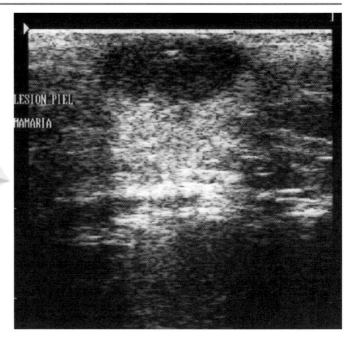

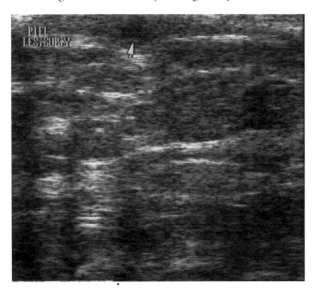

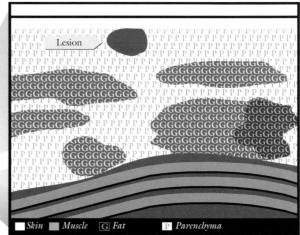

Fig. 4.53 Image of a suppurating lesion on the skin which occupies only a superficial area, without compromising the gland.

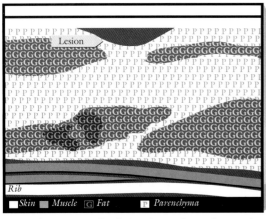

Fig. 4.54 Image of a lesion located on the areolar border which was diagnosed as suppuration of one of the accessory glands of the areola.

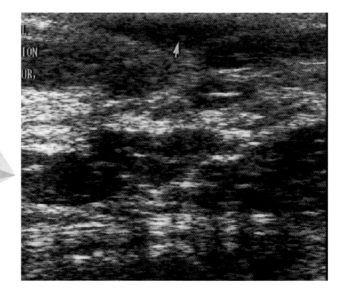

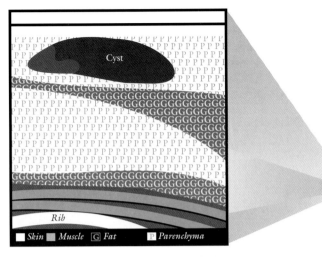

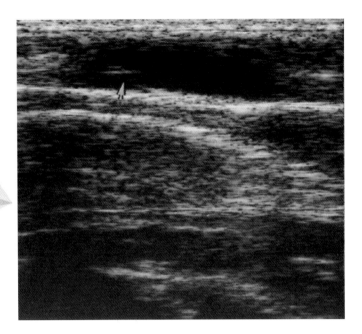

Fig. 4.55 Image of a hypoechoic lesion displaying small echoes in one sector which is in contact with the skin but does not compromise the mammary parenchyma. It was diagnosed as a sebaceous cyst.

Other Benign Tumors

The breast is susceptible to lesions which affect the skin. These lesions are normally discovered by the patient or during a clinical examination. Ultrasound imaging is especially useful in these cases because its ability to determine depth often eliminates the need for invasive techniques.

The most common are:
- **Contagiosum molluscum.**
- **Condyloma acuminatum.**
- **Warts.**
- **Verrucoid nevus.**

The following brief outline gives the criteria by which tumors can be determined to be benign, including both characteristics inherent to the nodule and indirect features displayed by adjacent tissues.

1) Direct characteristics:
- Well-defined borders
- Regular margins.
- Elliptic shape.
- Large lobulations (one or two).
- Homogeneous internal echostructure.
- Enhancement around the borders of the tumor.
- Shadows, or lateral sonic attenuation.
- Diameter parallel to the skin greater than perpendicular diameter.

2) Indirect characteristics:
- Displacement of surrounding tissues.
- Unaltered subcutaneous tissue.
- Mobility and elasticity.

The following statistics regarding benign tumors were published by Stravros et al.:

(1) Hyperechogenicity presents a sensitivity and negative predictive value of 100%.

(2) One or two lobulations: sensitivity and negative predictive value of 99.2%

(3) Elliptic shape: sensitivity, 97.6%; and negative predictive value, 99.1%.

(4) Fine capsule: sensitivity, 95.2%, and negative predictive value, 98.8%.

These statistics suggest that combinations of the following parameters indicate benignity:
- **Internal uniform hyperechogenicity.**
- **Elliptic shape with an echogenic capsule.**
- **Large lobulations with an echogenic capsule.**
- **No sign indicative of malignancy.**

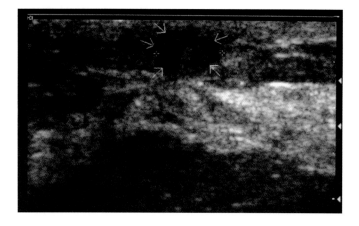

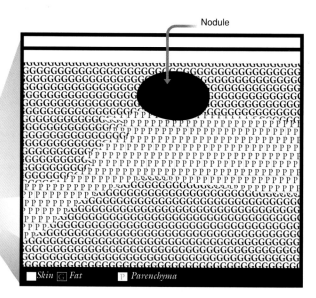

Fig. 4.56 Image of a small, hypoechoic nodule in contact with the superficial layers of the skin in a patient complaining of a palpable nodule. Diagnosed as an inflammatory process of the Montgomery's glands.

References

- Rosen PP, Cantrell B, Muller DL, *et al.:* Juvenile papillomatosis (Swiss cheese disease) of the breast. *Am J Surg Pathol* 1980; 4:3-12.
- Rosen PP: Papillary duct hyperplasia of the breast in children and young adults. *Cancer,* 1985; 56:1611-1617.
- Kersschot EA, Hermans ME, Pauwels C *et al.:* Juvenile paillomatosis of the breast. Sonographic appearance. *Radiology* 1988; 169:631-633.
- Cole-Beuglet C, Soriano R, Kurt A *et al.:* Ultrasound, X-ray mamography and histopathology of cystocarcinoma phylloides. *Radiology,* 1983; 146:481-486.
- Mourou MY, Pujol J, Lamarque JL: La tumeur Phyllode du sein. Approche diagnostique. Bilan actuel. *J Le Sein,* 1992; 2:9-15.
- Jackson VP: The role of US in breast imaging. *Radiology,* 1990; 177:305-311.
- Adler DD: Ultrasound of benign breast conditions. *Semin Ultrasound CT MR,* 1989; 10:106-118.
- Moskowitz M: Circumscribed lesions of the breast. In: Moskowitz M, ed.: *Syllabus: a diagnostic categorical course in breast imaging.* Oak Brook, III Radiological Society of North America, 1986; 31-33.
- Jokich PM, Monticciolo DL, Adler YT: Breast ultrasonography. *Radiol Clin North Am,* 1992; 30:993-1009.
- Jakson VP, Rothschild PA, Kreipe DL *et al.:* The spectrun of sonographic findings of fibroadenoma of the breast. *Invest Radiol,* 1986; 21:34-40.
- Cole-Beuglet C, Soriano RZ, Kurtz AB, Goldberg BB: Fibroadenoma of the brreast: sonomammography correlated with pathology in 122 patients. *AJR,* 1983; 140:369-375.
- Bassett LW, Ysrael M, Gold RH, Ysrael C: Usefulness of mammography and sonography in women les than 35 years old. *Radiology* 1991; 180:831-835.
- Hilton SW, Leopolod GR, Olson LK, Wilson SA: Real-time breastsonography application in 300 consecutive patients. *AJR,* 1986; 147:479-486.
- Vlaisavljevic: Differentation of solid breast tumors on the basis of their primary echographic characterristics as revealed by real-time scanning of the uncompressed breast. *Ultrasound Med Biol,* 1988; 14 (suppl 1):59-73.
- Hackeloer B-J, Duda V, Lauth G: *Ultrasound Mammography.* Springer-Verlag, New York, 1989.
- Jackson VP, Rothschild PA, Kreipke DL *et al.:* The spectrum sonographic findings of fibroadenoma of the breast. *Invest Radiol,* 1986; 34-40.
- Formage BD, Lorigan JG, Andry E: Fibroadenoma of the breast: sonographic appearane. *Radiology,* 1989; 172:671-675.
- Cole-Beuglet C, Soriano RZ, Kurtz, AB, Goldberg, BB: Fibroadenoma of the breast: sonomammography correlated with pathology in 122 patients. *AJR,* 1983; 140:369-375.
- Moran CS: Fibroadenoma of the breast during pregnancy and lactation. *Arch Surg,* 1935; 31:688-708.
- Kopans DB, Meyer JE, Proppe KH: Ultrasonographic, xeromammographic and histologic correlation of a fibroadenolipoma of the breast. *J Clin Ultrasound,* 1982; 10:409-411.
- Adler DD, Jeffries DO, Helvie MA: Sonographic features of breast hamartomas. *J Ultrasound Med,* 1990; 9:85-90.
- Spalding JE: Adeno-lipoma and lipoma of the breast. *Guy's Hosp Rep,* 1945; 94: 80-84.
- Strickles EA, Filly RA, Callen PW: Benign breast lesions: ultrasound detection and diagnosis. *Radiology,* 151: 1984; 467-470.
- Byrd BF, Hartmann, WH, Graham LS, Hogle HH: Mastopathy in insulin-dependent diabetes. *Ann Surg,* 205: 1987; 529-532.
- Gartstin WIH, Aufmann ZK, Michell MJ, Baum M: Fibrous mastopathy in insulin dependent diabetes. *Clin Radio* 1991, 44: 89-91.

5

Solid Malignant Nodule

M. E. Lanfranchi

Introduction

Statistics show that breast cancer affects more women than any other type of cancer. In the U.S. only skin cancer is more frequent, and in developing countries it is the third most frequent cancer, after cancers of the cervix and the stomach.

The most recent comparative study, conducted between 1985 and 1989, examined incidences of cancer in 137 different population groups in 36 countries (those which keep statistical records of cancers).

Table 5.1 below shows the incidence of cancer per 100,000 women ages 35 to 64.

Country	Rate*
U.S.A.	
Caucasian women	187.3
Black women	138.3
Hawaii	
Caucasian women	211.0
Japanese women	140.2
Chinese women	165.7
Canada (Alberta)	150.4
Italy (Florence)	149.6
Sweden	133.8
Great Britain	123.5
Finland	116.1
Belarus	62.8
Costa Rica	58.4
India (Bombay)	55.3
Japan (Osaka)	53.8
China (Shanghai)	49.9

Table 5.1

*Rates are calculated every 100.000 women.

Notably, the incidence of breast cancer in American and European women is two to three times that of women from Asian countries such as China and Japan. However, Asian women who have immigrated to the U.S. and Hawaii show nearly the same rates of cancer as American women, which suggests the importance of environmental factors in breast cancer.

The American Cancer Society estimates that each year approximately 182,000 new cases of invasive cancer, and 25,000 cases of ductal or lobular carcinomas *in situ* will be diagnosed. In 1995 alone 46,000 women died of this disease, at a rate of 126 per day. Unfortunately, there is still no effective way to prevent this disease, thus the strategy for fighting it relies on early detection followed by adequate treatment.

Figure 5.1 below shows the number of both cases and deaths from breast cancer between 1980 and 1995.

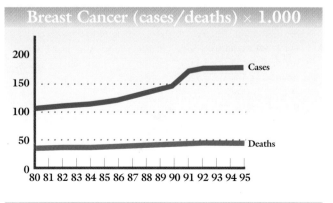

Figure 5.1

Table 5.2 shows statistics compiled by the American Cancer Society between 1979 and 1991 which give the percentage of breast cancers affecting 7 different age groups. As the table demonstrates, diagnosis of breast cancer before age 25 is quite rare (less than 0.3%). The rate increases rapidly between 39 and 49 years of age, more than doubling every 5 years. The rate slows between 50-59 years of age, corresponding to the period during which

Age	% of the Total
20-29	0.3
30-39	4.6
40-49	18.6
50-59	15.6
60-69	22.7
70-79	24.3
80 and more	13.9
All ages	100

Table 5.2

most women undergo menopause, only to rise again between 60-79 years of age.

Between 1980-1987 the rate of breast cancers increased greatly. It is not entirely clear if this is due to an actual increase in incidences of the disease, or if it is due to an increase in the number of screenings performed.

A study by White et al. suggests that increased screenings cannot completely explain the rise in diagnoses of cancer because all age groups showed a similar increase, not only the age group most often screened, women between the ages of 55 and 64.

On the other hand, screening explains the increase since 1980 in the rate of *in situ* and Stage 1 carcinomas. Interestingly, *in situ* carcinomas in caucasian women increased twice as much as those in black women, while Stage 1 carcinomas increased at the same rate for both races.

The five year survival rate for all stages of breast cancer is favorable, 83.1% and higher, depending on the timeliness of diagnosis.

The survival rate for breast cancer depends upon a number of factors: the stage at which it is discovered, the availability and quality of treatment, and the individual characteristics of the patient. In women it is the primary cause of premature death, followed by accidents, cardiac diseases, and suicide.

A number of risk factors have been determined by epidemiological analysis, such as:

- Early menarche.
- Late menopause.
- Nulliparity.
- First pregnancy at a late age.
- Exposure to high doses of radiation.

- History of contralateral breast cancer.
- Family history of breast cancer (mother or sister).
- Residence in an urban area.
- Personal history of ovary or endometrium cancer.
- High socio-economic position.
- Diet containing a high level of animal fat.
- Obesity.
- Personal history of a benign proliferate lesion.

The majority of the risk factors carry a relative incidence rate of 3.0 or less. However, family history of breast cancer, in mother or sister, carries a relative incidence rate of 2.5 for each case. If both mother and sister have had the disease the rate climbs to 13.6, which translates to a +50% chance of contracting the disease.

Familiarity with all the risk factors allows one to identify patients who, because of their high risk of developing carcinomas, should be examined often and with all available diagnostic tools.

Mammographic screening is extremely valuable as a method for early detection of malignant tumors, reducing by 30% the mortality rate in women over 50 years of age who are diagnosed with non-palpable tumors.

Breast cancer in its early stages may display the following features:

- Microcalcifications.
- Destruction of tissues.
- Asymmetrical density.
- Nodule.
- Ductal pathology.

A full 50% of carcinomas of the breast are located in the upper-outer quadrant, because of its high concentration of lobules.

The frequency in other areas is: Upper-inner: 15%; Lower-outer: 10%; Lower-inner: 5%; retroareolar: 17%, massive carcinoma: 3%.

Ultrasound is necessary for thorough diagnosis in the following cases:

- Inconclusive mammographical examination.
- Radiologically dense breasts, or breasts with asymmetrical density.
- Palpable or mammographically visible nodule.
- Non-palpable or poorly defined nodule in mammography.
- Nodule in a pregnant patient.
- Bloody discharge from the nipple, and/or determination of ductal pathology.
- Palpable nodule, not detected by mammography.

The results of a number of studies demonstrate the importance of ultrasound in the diagnosis of carcinomas. According to C. Hirst et al., 10% of carcinomas are non-palpable and undetectable by mammography. A study by Gordon and Goldenberg found that of 1,575 solid masses detectable only by ultrasound, 44 were carcinomas (2.8%), 16 of which were multifocal.

A study published by Cahill et al. studied 323 women with clinically diagnosed cancers and found that 9.3% had negative mammographies.

A similar study by Eideken et al. documented 499 women with breast cancer, 22% of which had no lesions detectable by mammography.

Wallis et al. published findings which state that 8.6% of carcinomas are not radiologically detectable.

An article by Kalisher has stated that nearly 50% of cancers not detectable by mammography occur in radiologically dense breasts.

A study conducted in 1995 by Dershaw et al. examined cases of radilogically dense brests. The study involved 114 women who were examined by ultrasound; 78% of the women were under 50 years of age, and of these 88% were found to have radiologically dense breasts. Within this group 20 cysts and 7 cancers were found which were not detectable by mammography.

It is worth noting here that only between 10% and 30% of masses detected by mammography or palpatation are found to be cancers.

Due to the difficulty of detecting microcalcifications by sonography even an ultrasound study which reveals no nodules or lesions does not rule out the possibility of cancer. Ultrasound can only evaluate microcalcifications which are located within nodules or masses, or those of a relatively large size. It cannot be used to evaluate microcalcifications isolated in the parenchyma.

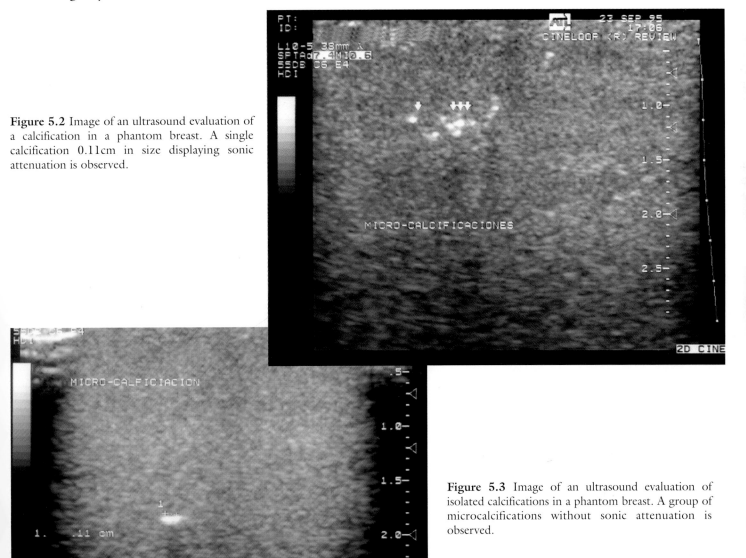

Figure 5.2 Image of an ultrasound evaluation of a calcification in a phantom breast. A single calcification 0.11cm in size displaying sonic attenuation is observed.

Figure 5.3 Image of an ultrasound evaluation of isolated calcifications in a phantom breast. A group of microcalcifications without sonic attenuation is observed.

WHO Classification

In 1981 the World Health Organization published the following guidelines for the classification of cancers:

I *Epithelial Tumors*
  1. Non-invasive carcinoma:
   -Intraductal.
   -Lobular *in situ.*

  2. Invasive carcinoma:
   -Invasive ductal (includes all non-specific carcinomas)
   -Invasive ductal with a predominant intraductal component.
   -Invasive lobular.
   -Mucinous.
   -Medular.
   -Papillary ductal.
   -Tubular.
   -Adenocystic.
   -Secretory (juvenile).
   -Adenocarcinoma with apocrine metaplasia.
   -Carcinoma with metaplasia (squamous, cartilaginous, bone, etc.).
   -Other carcinomas (lipid secretory, carcinoid, etc.)

  3. Paget's carcinoma of the nipple

II. *Mixed tumors, involving epithelial and conjuctive tissue*
   -Malignant phyllodes tumor.

Clinical States of Breast Cancer (TNM)

T Classification

Tx	Impossible to determine the size of the primary tumor.
Tx	Non-evident primitive tumor.
Tis	Carcinoma *in situ.* Clinical: Paget's disease of the nipple without palpable mass. Pathology: intraductal carcinoma, lobular carcinoma *in situ* or Paget's disease without an invasive component.
T1	Tumor of 2 cm or less in diameter at its largest point.
	- **T1a:** 0.5 cm or less.
	- **T1b:** from 0.5 to 1 cm.
	- **T1c:** from 1 to 2 cm.
T2	Tumor between 2 and 5 cm in diameter at its largest point.
T3	Tumor more than 5 cm in diameter at its largest point.
T4	Tumor of any size, extending towards the thoracic wall (including ribs, serratus major and intercostals, not the pectoralis major) and/or skin.
	- **T4a:** extension towards the thoracic wall.
	- **T4b:** edema or ulceration of the skin or nodules.
	- **T4c:** both.
	- **T4d:** inflammatory carcinoma.

Table 5.3

N Classification

Clinical classification

Nx	Indefinite regional lymph nodes (previously excised).
N0	Absence of metastasical lymph nodes.
N1	Metastasis in mobile homolateral axillary lymph nodes.
N2	Metastasis in fixed homolateral lymph nodes.
N3	Metastasis in the lymph nodes of the homo-lateral internal mammarian chain.

Pathological Classification

Nx	Indefinite regional lymph nodes.
N0	Axillary lymph nodes free from metastasis.
N1	Metastasis in mobile homolateral axillary lymph nodes:
	- **N1a:** Micrometastasis (not more than 0.2 cm)
	- **N1b:** Metastasis of more than 2 cm.
	- **N1b1:** Metastasis in one to three lymph nodes between 0.2 and 2 cm.
	- **N1b2:** Metastasis in four or more lymph nodes between 0.2 and 2 cm.
	- **N1b3:** Metastasis of less than 2 cm with a broken capsule.
	- **N1b4:** Metastasis larger than 2 cm.
N2	Metastasis in fixed homolateral axillary lymph nodes.
N3	Homolateral metastasis of the internal mammary lymph node chain.

Table 5.4

M Classification

Mx	No distant metastasis can be determined.
M0	Without distant metastasis.
M1	Distant metastasis (includes metastasis to homolateral supra-clavicular lymph nodes)

Table 5.5

G Classification
Histological degree

Gx	Indeterminate degree of differentiation.
G1	Well-differentiated.
G2	Moderately differentiated.
G3	Poorly differentiated.
G4	Undifferentiated.

Table 5.6

Classification by Stages

Stage	T	N	M
0	Tis	N0	M
1	T1	N0	M0
11a	T0	N1	M0
	T1	N1	M0
	T2	N0	M0
11B	T2	N1	M0
	T3	N0	M0
111a	T0	N2	M0
	T1	N2	M0
	T2	N2	M0
	T3	N1-2	M0
111b	T4	Any T	M0
	Any T	N3	M0
IV	Any T	Any T	M1

Table 5.7

Ultrasound Evaluation

Ultrasound measurements of tumor size and volume have been proved accurate by comparison with the actual nodules after excision. In cases of central tumors in voluminous breasts, or tumors which have caused a reaction in neighboring tissues, palpation may lead to an overestimation of tumor size. Therefore, ultrasound evaluation is an important counterpart to clinical evaluation because it is the only diagnostic tool which can give accurate information on actual tumor volume.

Malignant Tumors in Ultrasound

Ultrasound is very reliable in cases involving solid nodules. However, due to its high sensitivity and low specificity it is less effective in cases of carcinomas located inside cysts or ducts. For example, in many cases ultrasound is unable to distinguish between intracystic or intracanicular papilloma and similarly located carcinomas.

I. Solid Nodule

1) Solid Homogeneous Tumor with an Irregular Border

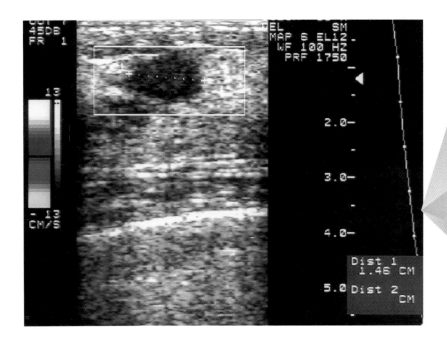

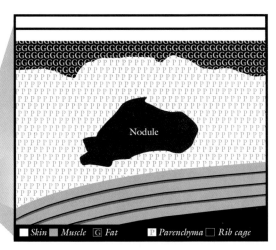

Figure 5.4 Image of a solid nodule 14 x 19mm in size with defined borders, homogeneous echoes, and an irregularity in one sector. Biopsy showed a mucinous carcinoma.

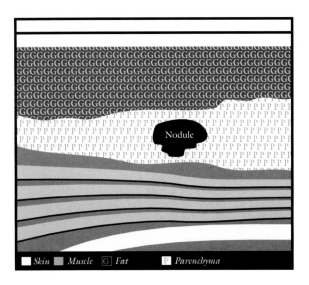

Figure 5.5 Image of a solid, hypoechoic nodule with irregular borders, 4 x 8mm in size, located in the parenchyma of the upper-outer quadrant of the breast. Carcinoma.

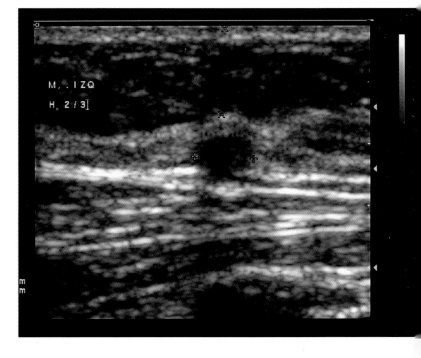

2) *Solid Homogeneous Tumor with Irregular Borders*

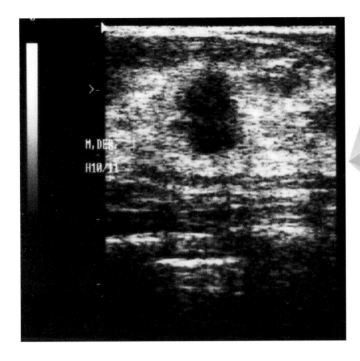

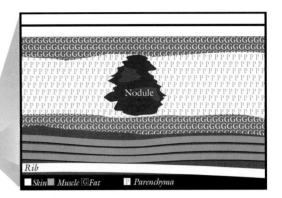

Figure 5.6 Image of a solid, non-palpable nodule with irregular borders in a 51 year-old patient with radiologically dense breasts. The nodule is approximately 9mm in diameter with the largest area perpendicular to the skin. Histological results confirmed an infiltrating lobular carcinoma with metastasis in one of the lymph nodes.

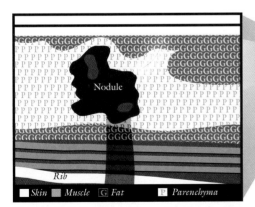

Figure 5.7 Image of a solid, hypoechoic nodule with irregular borders, faint posterior sonic attenuation and displaying echogenic reaction in the adjacent tissues. A biopsy confirmed it to be a carcinoma.

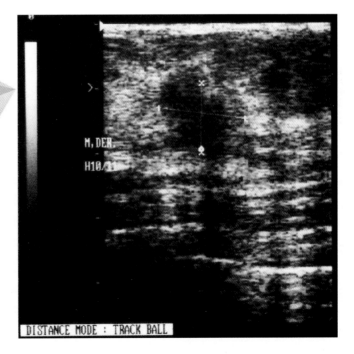

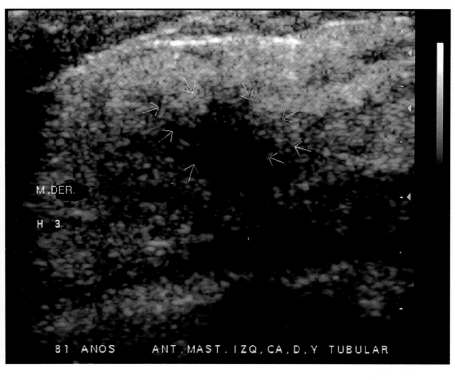

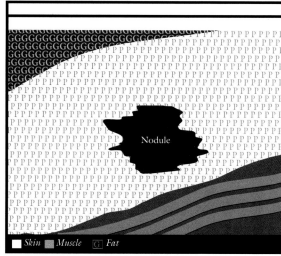

Skin ▢ Muscle G Fat

Figure 5.8 Image of a hypoechoic nodule with completely irregular borders and posterior attenuation in an 81 year-old patient with a prior mastectomy two years before due to invasive ductal carcinoma with areas of tubular carcinoma. This nodule was located in the upper-outer quadrant of the breast and was diagnosed as a carcinoma.

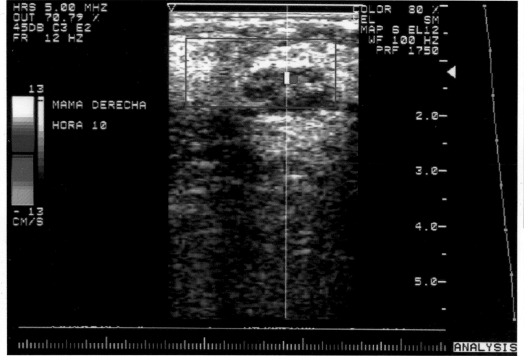

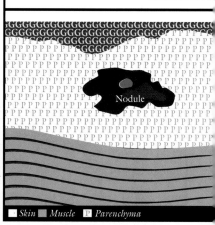

▢ Skin ▢ Muscle P Parenchyma

Figure 5.9 Image of a nodule with irregular borders and heterogeneous echostructure, 15 x 8mm in size, in a 44 year-old patient. This image shows that the nodule contains a vessel. Infiltrating ductal carcinoma.

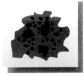

3) Solid Heterogeneous Tumor with Irregular Borders

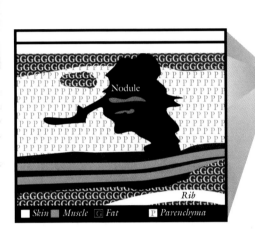

Figure 5.10 Image of a solid nodule with spiculated and completely irregular borders and sonic attenuation.

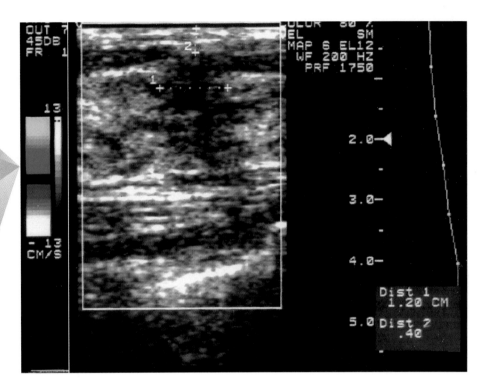

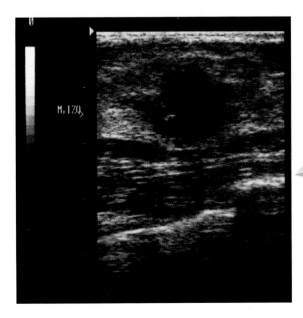

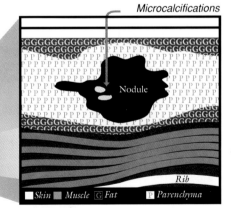

Figure 5.11 Image of a solid, hypoechoic nodule which has irregular borders and displays both a small calcification and lateral prolongations. Biopsy-proven carcinoma.

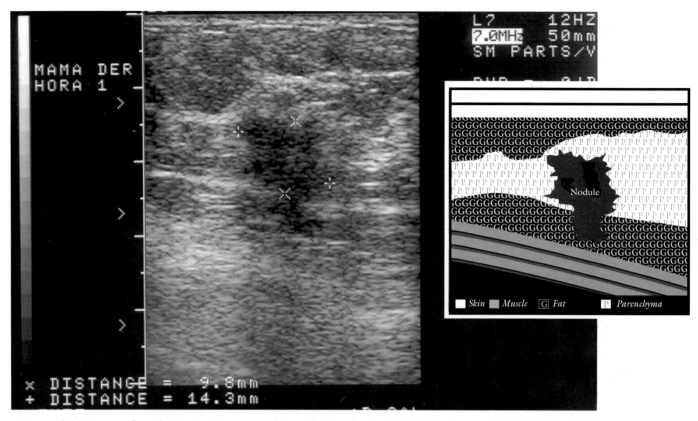

Figure 5.12 Image of a solid, heterogeneous nodule with irregular borders. The axis perpendicular to the skin is predominant, a sign of neoplasy. Infiltrating ductal carcinoma.

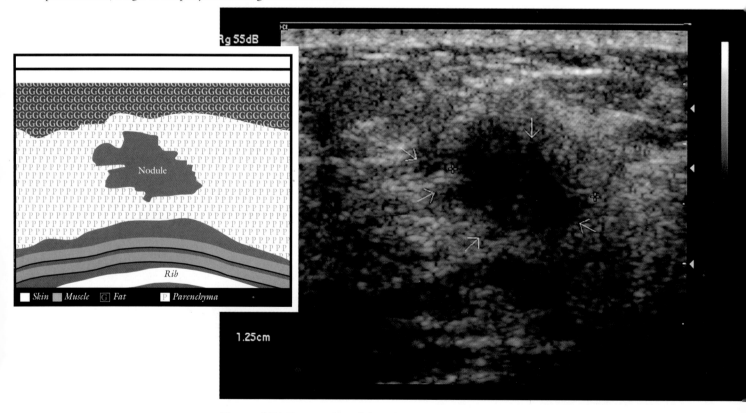

Figure 5.13 Image of a solid nodule 12mm in diameter which has completely irregular borders, two lateral prolongations and displays signs of branching in a patient complaining of increased tension in the left breast. Histopathology confirmed an intraductal carcinoma.

4) *Solid Heterogeneous Tumor with Irregular Borders and Areas of Necrosis or Hemorrhage*

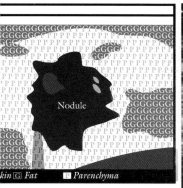

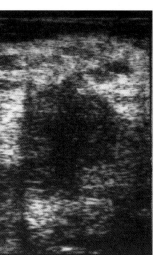

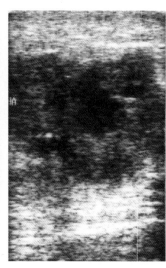

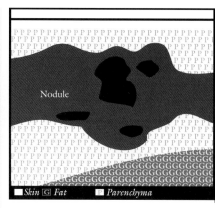

Figure 5.14 Image of a solid nodule completely heterogeneous echostructure, irregular borders and spicules. tal carcinoma.

Figure 5.15 Image of a nodule with irregular borders, heterogeneous echostructure, and a central hypoechoic area consistent with necrosis. Diagnosed as a carcinoma.

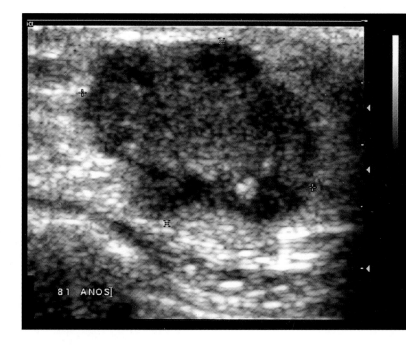

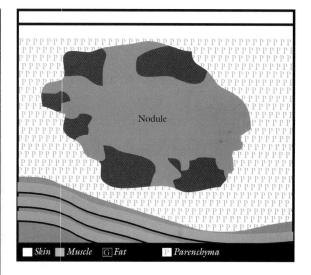

Figure 5.16 Image of a hypoechoic mass, 20 x 15mm in size, with completely irregular and heterogeneous borders, calcifications, and areas of lower echogenicity due to necrosis in an 81 year-old patient complaining of a painless, palpable nodule. The tumor involves all the mammary layers without reaching the retromammary fat. The histological evaluation confirmed an invasive ductal carcinoma with a high degree of anaplasia, a moderate mitotic rate, and marked vascular and lymphatic invasion.

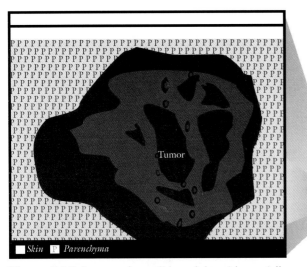 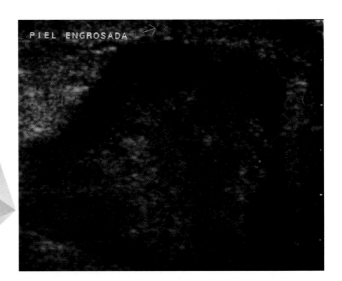

Figure 5.17 Image of a solid nodule with partially defined borders and heterogeneous echostructure in a patient complaining of a painful, palpable nodule and thickening of the skin. Histopathology showed an invasive ductal carcinoma.

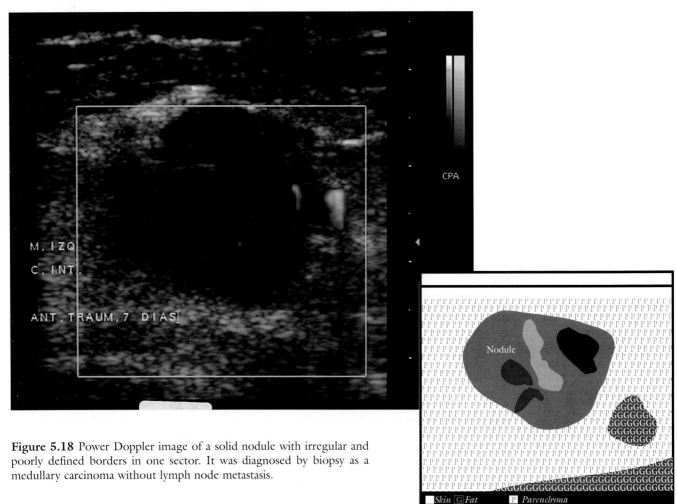

Figure 5.18 Power Doppler image of a solid nodule with irregular and poorly defined borders in one sector. It was diagnosed by biopsy as a medullary carcinoma without lymph node metastasis.

5) Solid Heterogeneous Tumor with Irregular Borders and Partial Posterior Acoustic Shadowing

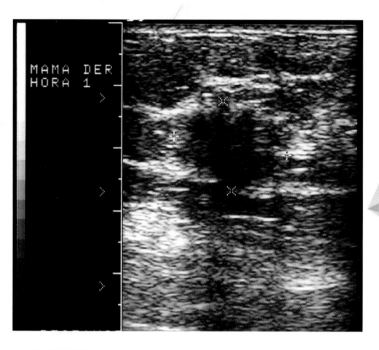

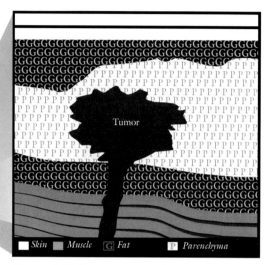

Figure 5.19 Image of a nodule 14 x 9mm in size with completely irregular borders, heterogeneous echostructure, and slight sonic attenuation. Carcinoma.

6) Solid Heterogeneous Tumor with Irregular Borders and Complete Posterior Acoustic Shadowing

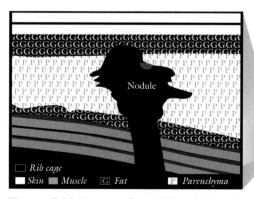

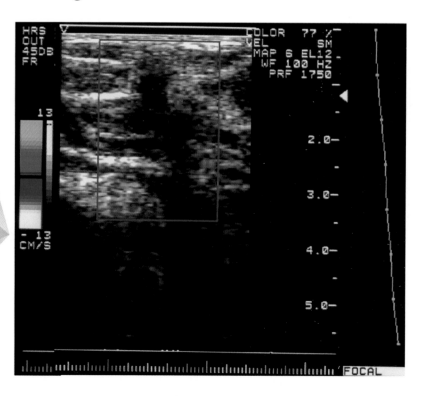

Figure 5.20 Image of a solid nodule with completely irregular borders, spicules, and partial posterior sonic attenuation. The surrounding tissues display alteration and an irregular increase in echogenicity. The nodule was diagnosed as an infiltrating ductal carcinoma with an invasion of the subcutaneous cell tissue.

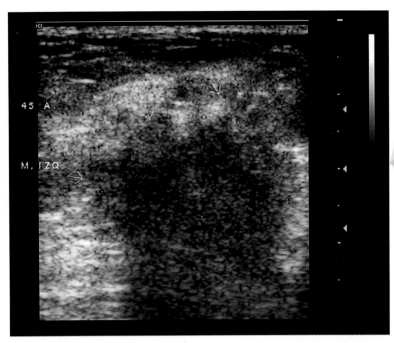

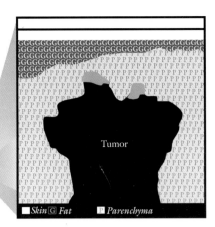

Figure 5.21 Image of a solid nodule, 26mm in diamete with completely irregular borders, sonic attenuation spicules, and areas of echogenic crown due to invasion o desmoplastic reaction of the subcutaneous tissue. The nodu is located in the upper-outer quadrant of the left breast of 45 year-old patient and its longest axis is parallel to the ski Histological examination showed an infiltrating duct carcinoma with multiple lymph node metastasis. Treatmer involved mastectomy and axillary emptying.

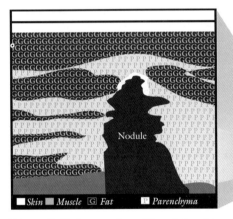

Figure 5.22 Image of a solid nodule with irregular borders. An infiltrating ductal carcinoma was diagnosed.

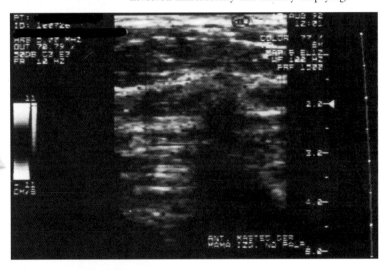

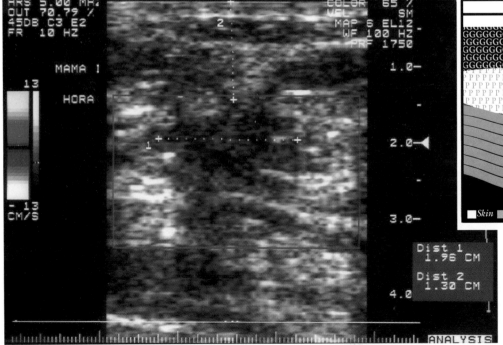

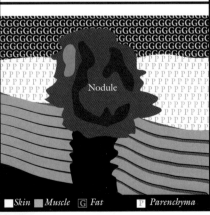

Figure 5.23 Image of a solid, heterogeneous nodule which involves the subcutaneous tissue and induces complete posterior sonic shadowing. Carcinoma.

7) Tumor Limited to the Parenchyma

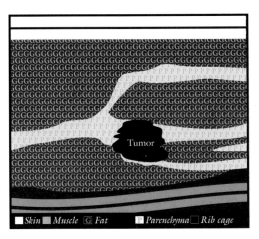

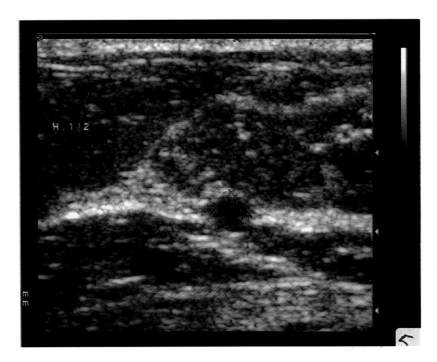

Figure 5.24 Image of a solid, hypoechoic nodule with irregular borders, 0.37cm in size and located at a depth of 15mm from the skin in a breast with considerable fatty infiltration. It is an *in situ* lobular carcinoma with peripheral areas of sclerosing adenosis.

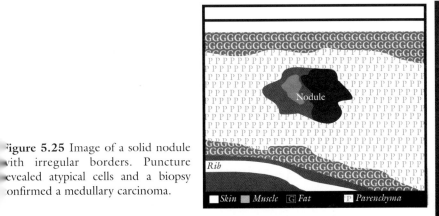

Figure 5.25 Image of a solid nodule with irregular borders. Puncture revealed atypical cells and a biopsy confirmed a medullary carcinoma.

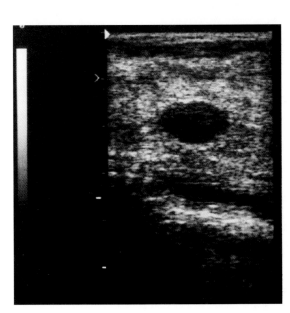

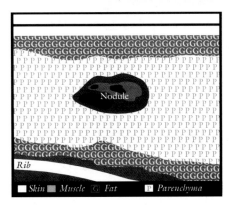

Figure 5.26 See Figure 5.23

8) *Tumor Compromising the Superficial Layers*

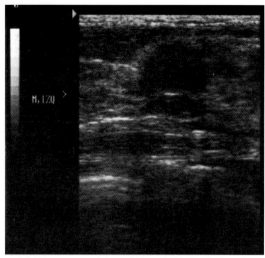

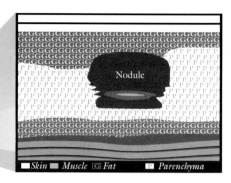

Skin · *Muscle* · G *Fat* · P *Parenchyma*

Figure 5.27 Image of a solid nodule 14 x 16mm in size. The largest diameter is perpendicular to the skin and it displays an irregularity in the posterior area and spicules in the superficial area which modify the premammary fat. Histopathology showed a medullary carcinoma.

9) *Tumor Compromising the Deep Layers*

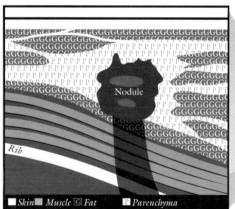

Skin · *Muscle* · G *Fat* · P *Parenchyma*

Figure 5.28 Image of a solid nodule with irregular borders, spicules, and discrete posterior sonic attenuation. Infiltrating ductal carcinoma.

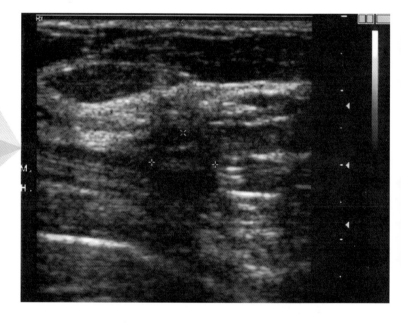

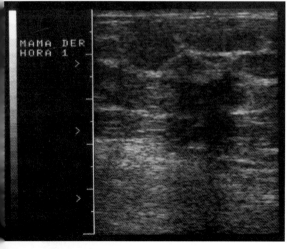

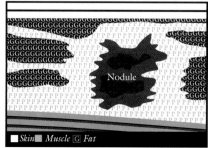

Skin · *Muscle* · G *Fat*

Figure 5.29 Image of a solid nodule with irregular borders. The parenchyma displays fatty infiltration and produces heterogeneous echoes. There is a hyperechogenic reaction in the surrounding tissues. The nodule was diagnosed as an infiltrating ductal carcinoma.

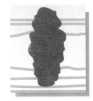

10) *Tumor Affecting All Layers*

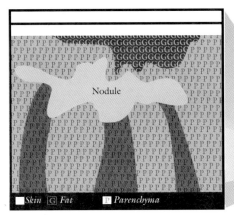

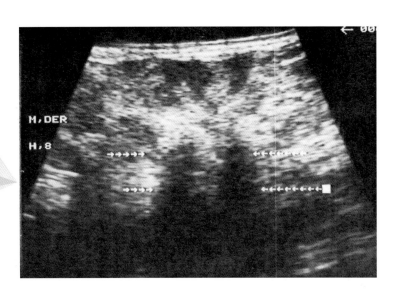

Figure 5.30 Image of a solid nodule which compromises all the mammary layers and displays poorly defined borders and heterogeneous echoes. It was diagnosed by puncture as a carcinoma; a histological study indicated it to be non-specific, scirrhous, and invasive.

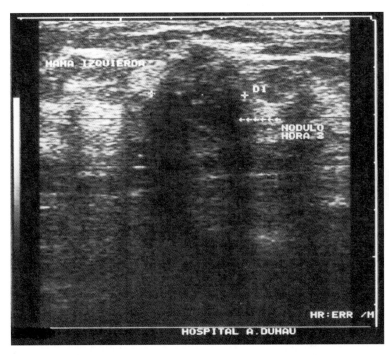

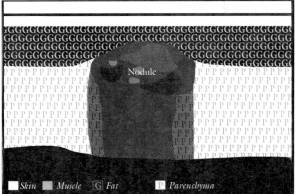

Figure 5.31 Image of a solid nodule with heterogeneous echostructure, partially defined borders, and considerable sonic attenuation in some sectors. Biopsy showed an infiltrating ductal carcinoma.

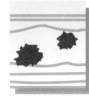

11) Multicentric Tumor

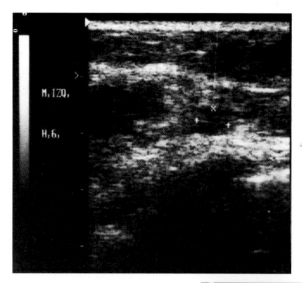

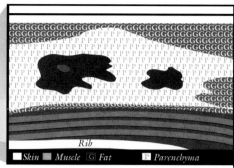

Figs. 5.32-5.34 Images of three nodules with similar characteristics: all are solid, displaying both low echogenicity and irregular borders. Biopsy confirmed a multicentric ductal carcinoma.

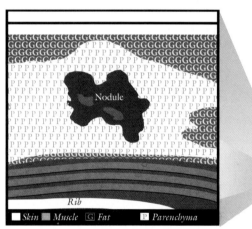

Figure 5.33 See above.

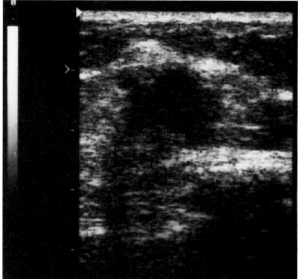

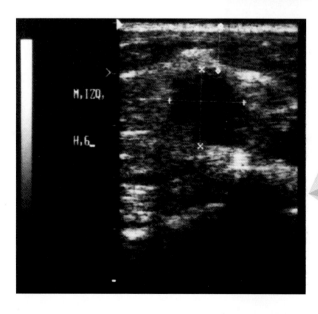

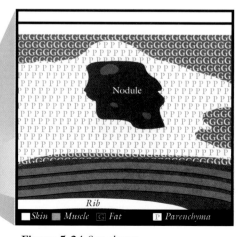

Figure 5.34 See above.

12) *Tumor with Axillary Metastasis*

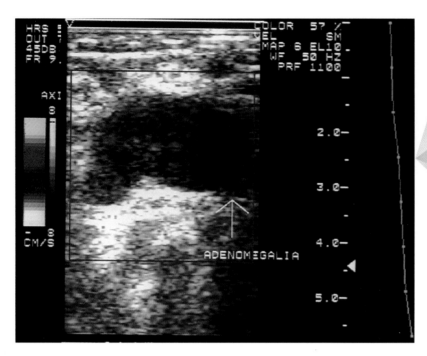

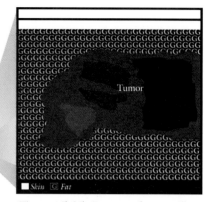

Figure 5.35 Image of an axillary mass composed of several large lymph nodes in close proximity, displaying irregular borders, lobulations, and heterogeneous echostructure. Metastatic invasion was diagnosed.

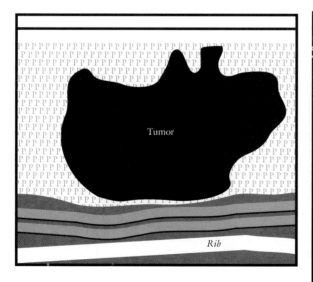

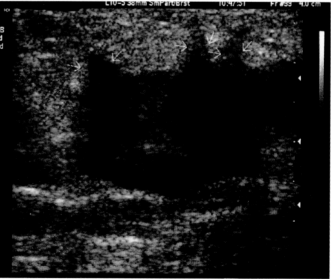

Figure 5.36.1 Image of a solid nodule which involves all the mammary layers but does not reach the retromammary fat. It displays irregular borders, spicules, and a number of prolongations caused by possible intraductal extension. Histopathology indicated an infiltrating ductal carcinoma with lymphatic and vascular invasion and a high degree of anaplasia.

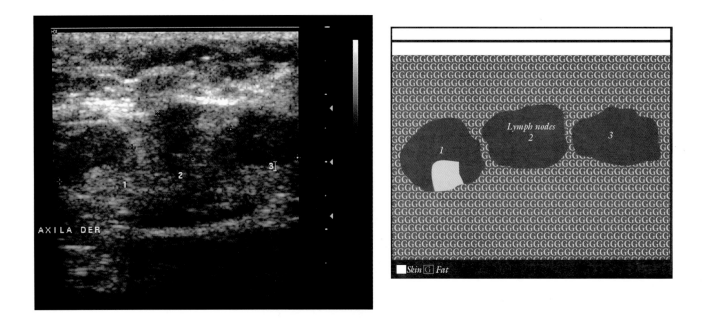

Figure 5.36.2 Image of three lymph nodes in the right axilla in close proximity; all three display irregular borders and a complete alteration in their echostructure. The first from the left displays an eccentric hilum, and the remaining two are hypoechoic and metastatic.

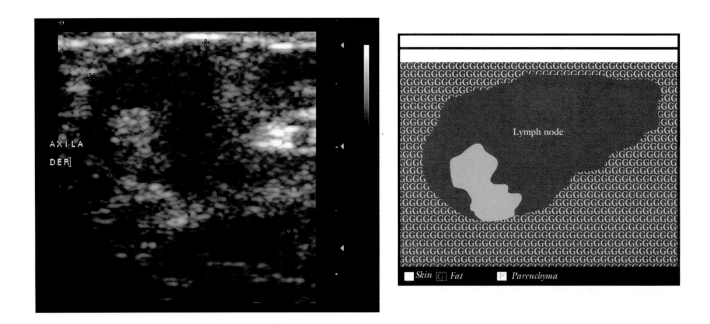

Figure 5.36.3 Lymph node with eccentric hilum from Figure 5.36.2 at greater magnification. The eccentric hilum is caused by an increase in thickness of the peripheral hypoechoic tissue in an area affected by partial metastatic invasion.

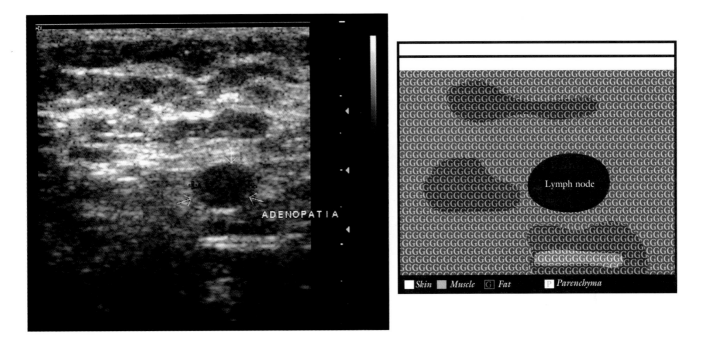

Figure 5.36.4 Image of a small lymph node 8 x 4mm in size which displays a decrease in echogenicity. The hilum cannot be identified. Metastasis was confirmed.

High resolution sonography has been used in an attempt to establish a correlation between ultrasound images of tumors and their histological types.

Invasive duct carcinoma is the most frequently encountered type, and it can be divided into three subgroups:

- **Scirrhous.**
- **Solid Tubular.**
- **Tubulopapillary.**

Scirrhous carcinoma generally has irregular borders, heterogeneous echoes, and significant sonic attenuation.

Solid, medullary, and mucoid tubular carcinmas are well-circumscribed masses which sometimes display posterior enhancement or lateral shadowing.

Tubulopapillary carcinoma can display any type of image, and cause alterations in neighboring tissues. In some cases these carcinomas may display interior microcalcifications.

Intraductal carcinoma can also be divided into three subgroups:

- **Circumscribed mass with homogeneous echoes.**
- **Poorly-defined mass with augmented echoes and its greatest diameter perpendicular to the skin.**
- **Ductal dilation.**

A study published by Eriko Tohno et al. studied 40 cases of various carcinomas (ductal, intraductal, *in situ* lobular and invasive) 11 of which did not display a nodular lesion detectable by ultrasound. These 11 cases were examined by mammography and revealed the following abnormalities: ductal dilation, solidified areas in dilated ducts, increases in glandular thickness, and distortion of ductal architecture with or without calcifications.

Another study performed by Ki Keuns Oh found 51 cases of bilateral carcinomas in a group of 1,399 cancers. These bilateral carcinomas were divided into two groups: synchronous, or those which appear simultaneously in both breasts; and metachronous, or those which appear at a later time in the contralateral breast.

The metachronous carcinomas commonly displayed ductal infiltration, and the average interval between appearance in each breast was 3.8 years. The average age of the patient was 43 years.

Multifocal carcinoma is a condition in which two or more carcinomas are found closer than 3 cm to one another in the same breast. The term multicentric is used when there are 2 or more carcinomas more than 3 cm apart.

As described in the first chapter, the image of a normal lymph node has the following characteristics:

- **An elongated or oval shape.**
- **A central area of greater echogenicity which corresponds to the hilum composed of adipose, conjunctive, and vascular tissues.**
- **A peripheral area of lower echogenicity composed of lymphatic tissue.**

When the lymph node is affected by metastasis it generally displays the following characteristics:

- **An irregular or rounded shape.**
- **Heterogeneous echostructure, with hypoechoic areas.**
- **The image of the hilum may be absent or partially obliterated.**
- **Areas of necrosis may be found.**
- **Metastatic adenopathy may have a pattern similar to that of a primitive breast tumor.**
- **Eccentric cortex hypertrophy (greater than 2 mm width).**

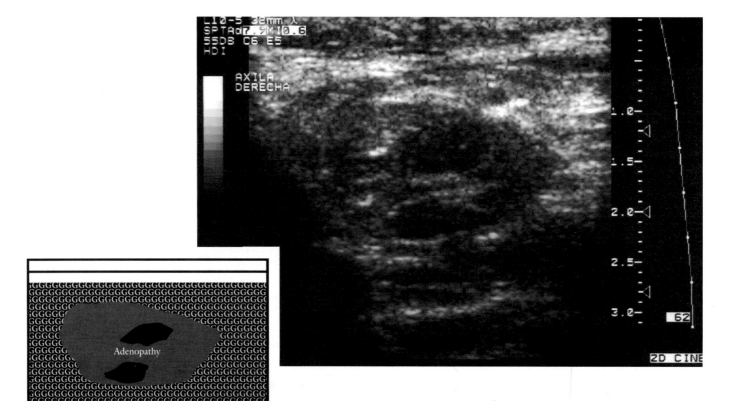

Figure 5.37 Image of a heterogeneous and hypoechoic axillary adenopathy, 38 x 21mm in size. Histopathology indicated metastatic invasion.

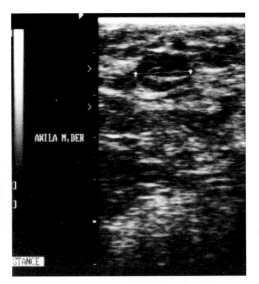

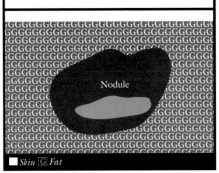

Figure 5.38 Image of a nodule located in the axilla displaying both low echogenicity and an eccentric echogenic area. A lymph node with an area of metastatic invasion was diagnosed.

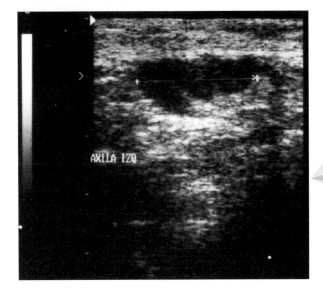

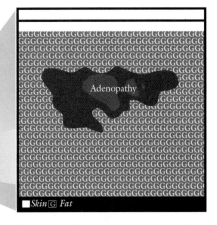

Figure 5.39 Image of an axillary nodule which was diagnosed as a metastatic adenopathy due to breast carcinoma.

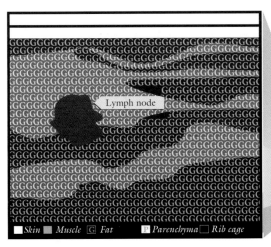

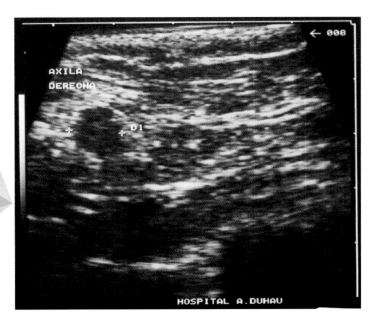

Figure 5.40 Image of a solid, hypoechoic nodule with irregular borders located in the axilla. The nodule was diagnosed as a metastatic lymph node.

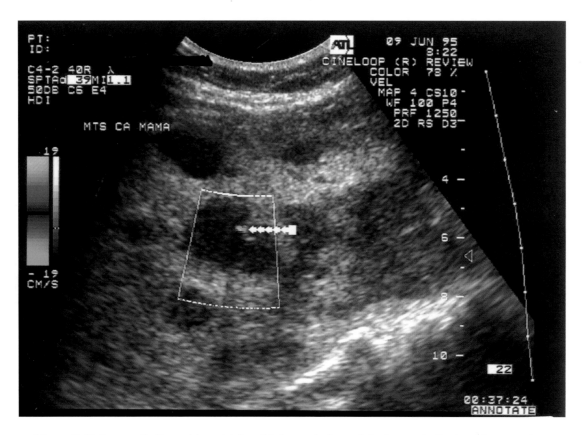

Figure 5.41 Image of a liver with multiple solid, hypoechoic, nodular images indicative of metastasis.

According to a study by Wei et al. the following statistics apply to the ultrasound diagnosis of carcinomas involving the lymph nodes: sensitivity: 84.1%, specificity: 97.1%, diagnostic accuracy: 92.1%, positive predictive value: 94.9%, and negative predictive value: 90.7%.

Metastasis in the hepatic parenchyma may be single or multiple, slightly hypoechoic and with well-defined but irregular borders.

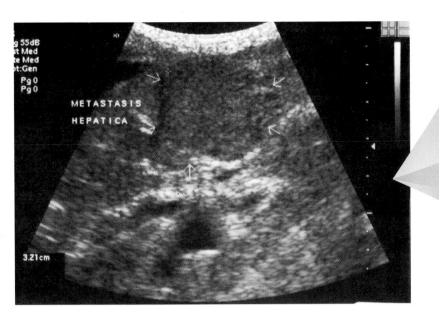

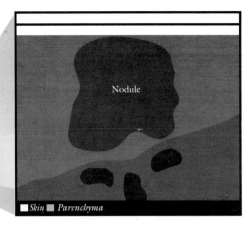

Figure 5.42 Image of a solid nodule within the hepatic parenchyma which displays an alteration of echogenicity and partially defined borders indicative of metastasis.

b) Intracystic Carcinoma

Although the incidence of intracystic carcinoma is low (0.5%), it should not be ruled out as a possibility.

Intracystic carcinoma, described in Chapter 3, may display various images, depending on the volume of the solid and liquid components of the cyst, as seen in the diagram below:

c) Carcinoma within a Duct

Intracanalicular carcinoma causes a dilation of the duct and in ultrasound images it appears as a mass within the duct itself. Longitudinal sections generally show the carcinoma following the path of the duct towards the nipple.

Intracystic Carcinomas.

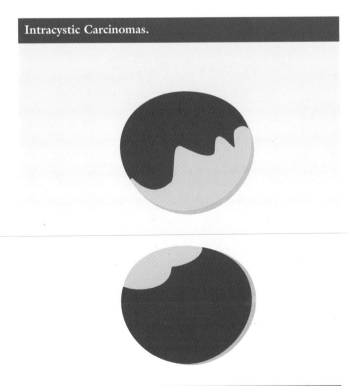

Figure 5.43

Carcinomas within a Duct.

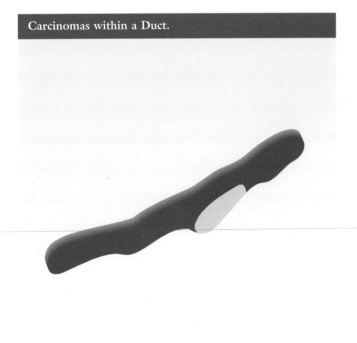

Figure 5.44

Other varieties of malignant tumors:
- **Inflammatory carcinoma.**
- **Leiomyosarcoma.**
- **Rhabdomyosarcoma.**
- **Angiosarcoma.**

- **Lymphosarcoma.**
- **Metastasis of other carcinomas** (for example, melanoma, rabdomyosarcoma, etc.)
- **Lymphomas.**
- **Skin tumors.**

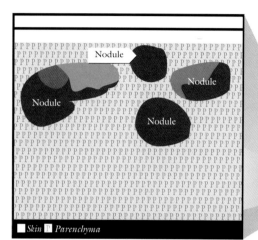

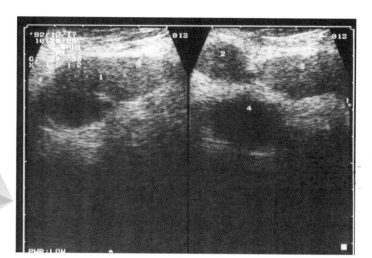

Figure 5.45 Image of multiple solid nodules of different sizes in the axillary tail of the breast. Metastasis from a melanoma.

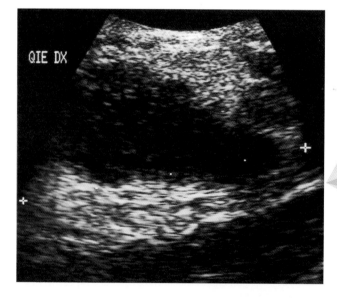

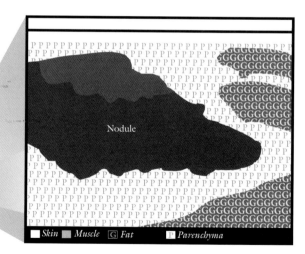

Figure 5.46 Image of a solid, palpable nodule with irregular borders. Biopsy showed a breast sarcoma. (Image courtesy of Dr. R. Rostagno)

Inflammatory carcinoma, as its name implies, generally presents with pain, inflammation, and an increase in breast volume, necessitating a differential diagnosis with mastitis. It represents 1.5% of all carcinomas, and may correspond to any of the of the histological types previously mentioned.

In addition to the characteristics of the tumor, inflammatory carcinoma is accompanied by a thickening of the skin, edema in all layers of the breast, and visible dilation of the subcutaneous lymph vessels.

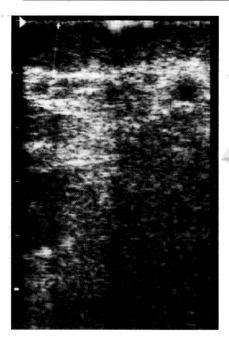

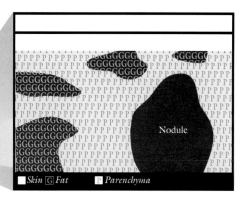

Figure 5.47 Image of a mass within the breast of a patient complaining of pain, sensations of heat, and inflammation. Image shows thickening of the skin and an area of alteration in the echogenicity which does not constitute a defined nodule. It was diagnosed by biopsy as an inflammatory carcinoma.

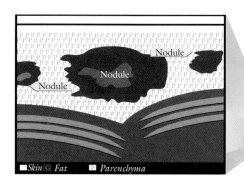

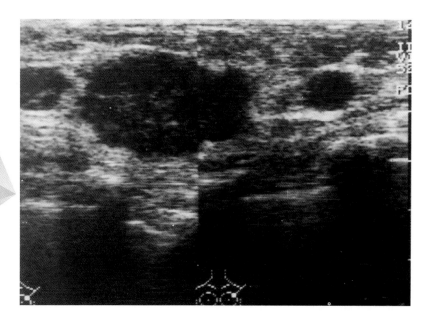

Figure 5.48 Image of three nodules of different sizes with irregular borders. Biopsy confirmed a carcinoma with metastasis located within the intramammary lymph nodes.

Thickening of the skin is a symptom which can accompany both benign and malignant pathologies. For this reason a detailed examination should be performed in order to establish a differential diagnosis.

The malignant pathologies which may provoke this symptom are:
- **Inflammatory carcinoma.**
- **Recurrence of carcinoma after conservative surgery.**
- **Lymphangitic carcinomatosis.**
- **Advanced breast metastasis.**
- **Breast carcinoma.**

The benign causes of this symptom are:
- **Acute mastitis.**
- **Traumatic injury and/or hematoma.**
- **Conservative surgery.**
- **Radiation treatments.**

Metastases found in the breast have an estimated prevalence of between 0.5 and 1.3%.

Clinically, metastasis may be single or multiple, generally mobile and with a rapid growth rate. The sonographic image is round, circumscribed, and usually without desmoplastic reaction. It can be difficult to distinguish from medullary, colloidal, and papillary tumors, which have a similar appearance. Between 8 and 25% of the cases of this pathology are bilateral.

Rhabdomyosarcoma, which can appear during adolescence, may produce this type of metastasis.

The incidence of lymphomas which originate in the breast is low, representing between 0.4% and 1.1% of all malignant tumors of the breast, and approximately 2.2% of extranodal tumors.

The majority of breast lymphomas are non-Hodgkin's, B-cell lymphomas (there are approximately 500 cases registered world-wide; 30% of which are registered in Japan). Thirty-five cases of this disease have been examined sonographically, 71% of which consisted of single, solid nodules with partially-defined and irregular borders. Some cases displayed posterior sonic attenuation, giving them a carcinoma-like appearance.

A study published by Meyer describes two types of breast lymphomas: follicular, which is practically identical to a carcinoma; and diffuse, which manifests itself as a swelling of the skin and a diffuse alteration of the gland.

An article by Collins et al. describes a case of multiple breast myeloma in a patient being treated for breast lymphoma. The ultrasound image displayed a solid mass with low echogenicity, and Doppler color revealed augmentation of the vascular signal.

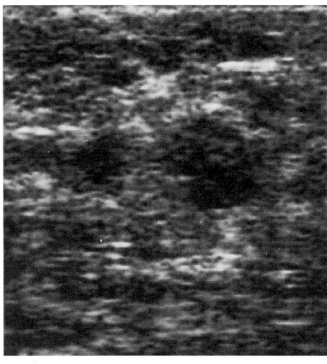

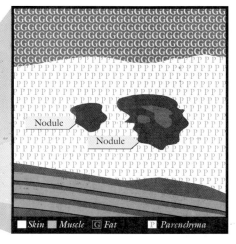

Figure 5.49 Image of two solid nodules of different sizes with irregular borders in close proximity to one another in patient with an antecedent of lymphoma. It was diagnosed by biopsy as a mammary lymphoma. (Image courtesy of Dr. R. Rostagno)

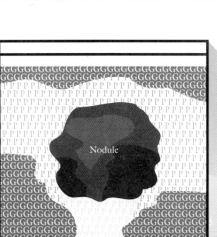

Figure 5.50 Image of a solid, hypoechoic nodule with irregular borders, heterogeneous echostructure and signs of neoplasia. Lymphoma.

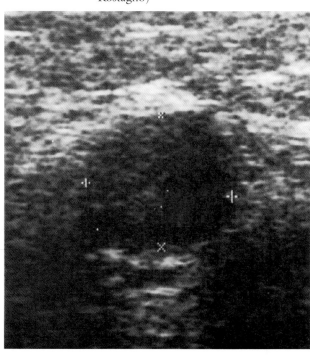

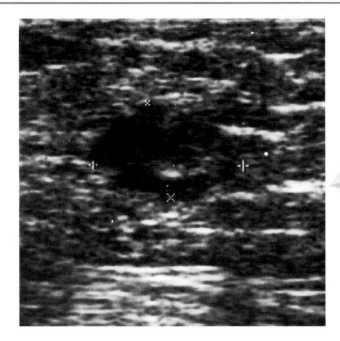

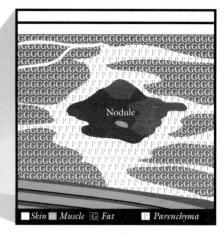

Figure 5.51 Image of a solid, hypoechoic, heterogeneous nodule with irregular borders located in a breast predominantly composed of fat. Lymphoma.

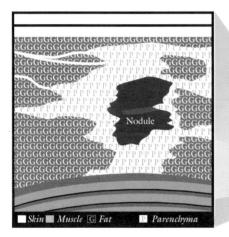

Figure 5.52 Image of a solid, hypoechoic, heterogeneous nodule with irregular borders. Lymphoma.

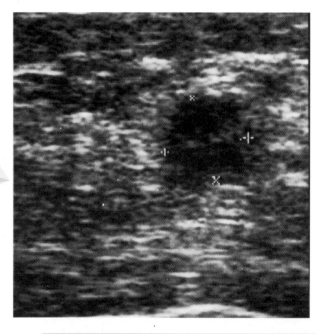

In summary, the **ultrasound criteria indicating malignancy** may be divided into:

1) **Direct Signs:** Those related to the tumor itself.
2) **Indirect Signs:** Those related to the tissues surrounding the tumor.

Tables 5.8 and 5.9 give the frequency of appearance of various direct and indirect signs.

Direct Signs	Frequency
Echostructure	
Heterogeneous	70%
Low echogenicity	52%
Homogeneous echoes	22%
Containing anechoic areas	9%
Containing hyperechogenic areas	5%
Borders	
Poorly-defined	89%
Spiculated	30%
Partially-defined	20%
Table 5.8	

Indirect Signs	Frequency
Posterior Acoustic Shadowing	
Central	75%
Partial	55%
Enhancement of the Posterior Wall	
Behind the tumor	10%
Behind part of the tumor	8%
Table 5.9	

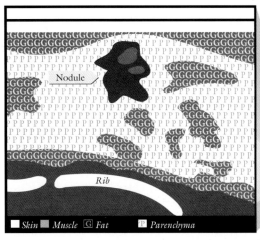

Figure 5.53 Image of a solid nodule 8 x 7mm in size displaying low echogenicity. Biopsy revealed atypical cells.

Depending upon its location, a tumor may modify the subcutaneous tissue, as described in Chapter 2 (see page 34).

Two common modifications are:

- **Disruption.**
- **Convergence.**

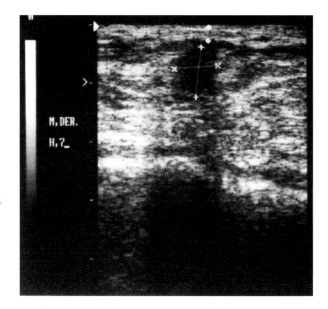

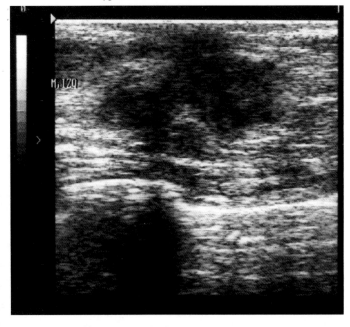

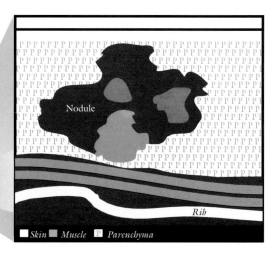

Figure 5.54 Image of a solid, heterogeneous, bilobulated nodule which has irregular borders and involves the superficial layers. Ductal carcinoma.

Table 5.10 shows the frequency of various histological types:

Pathology	Frequency
Infiltrating Ductal Carcinoma	**80%**
Infiltrating Lobular Carcinoma	**4%**
Medullary Carcinoma	**4%**
Mucous Carcinoma	**1.5%**
Metastasis	**1.5%**
DCIS	**4%**
Others	**5%**
Table 5.10	

Sonic attenuation is most common in tubular carcinomas and ductal carcinomas with a low degree of infiltration.

Angled margins and branching or spiculation have the greatest individual sensitivy and positive predictive value (PPV) for carcinoma.

The position of a lesion relative to the skin can be an important indicator of malignancy. The greatest diameter of most carcinomas is generally perpendicular to the skin, while in benign tumors the opposite is normally true.

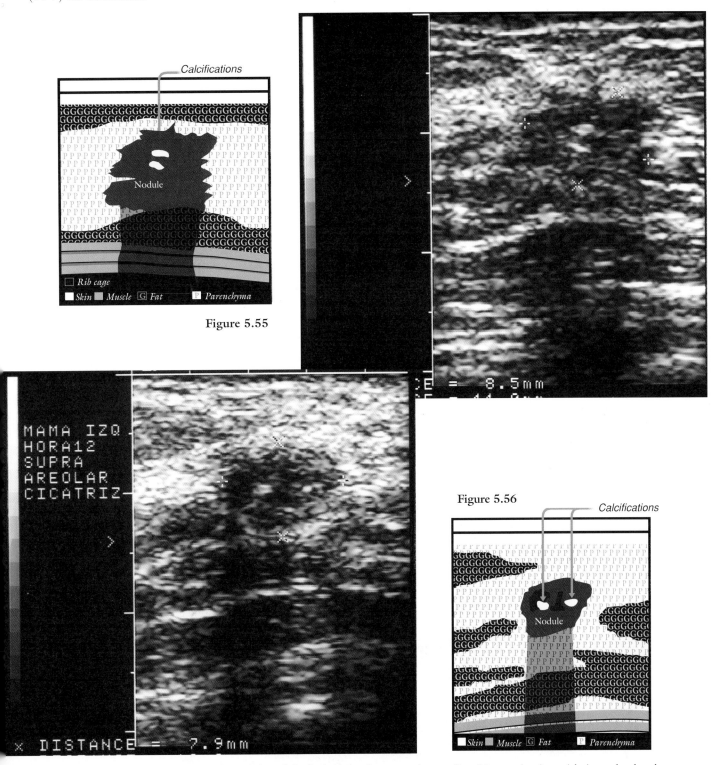

Figure 5.55

Figure 5.56

Figures 5.55-5.56 Two images of a solid nodule limited to the parenchyma, 8 x 11 mm in size with irregular borders, heterogenous echoes, and two calcifications in its interior. There is slight sonic attenuation behind the nodule. It was diagnosed as an infiltrating duct carcinoma.

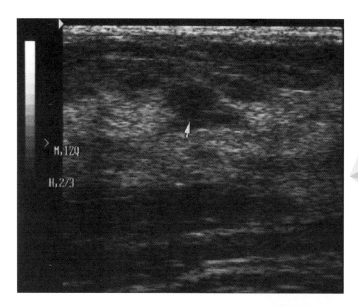

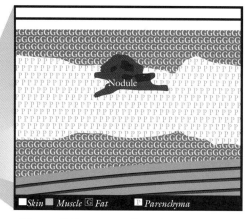

Figure 5.57 Image of a solid, non-palpable mass 7 x 4mm in size located on the anterior border of the parenchyma with spicules on the posterior side. Ductal carcinoma.

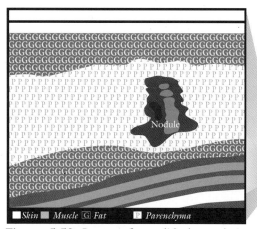

Figure 5.58 Image of a solid, hypoechoic, heterogeneous nodule with irregular borders and its largest diameter perpendicular to the skin. Infiltrating ductal carcinoma.

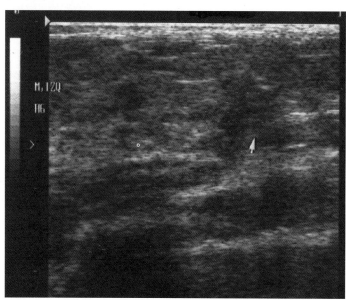

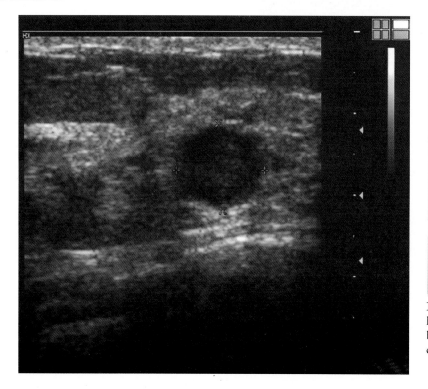

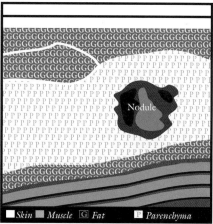

Figure 5.59 Image of a solid, heterogeneous nodule with irregular borders. It was diagnosed as a ductal carcinoma.

A prolongation of a tumor which involves a duct is referred to as a ductal extension. The most effective method of visualizing suspected ductal extensions is to perform radial explorations of the breast.

Approximately 70% of carcinomas appear heterogeneous in ultrasound; 30% of these heterogeneous carcinomas contain microcalcifications, which generally do not cause posterior acoustic shadow due to their small size.

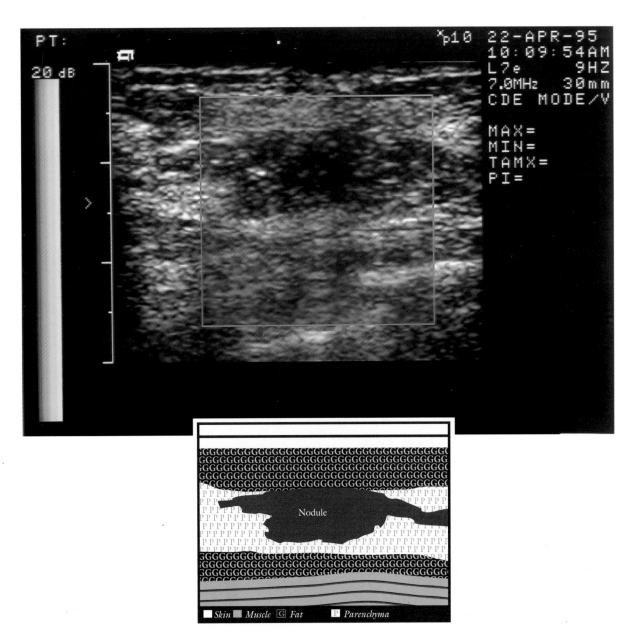

Figure 5.60 Image of a hypoechoic, heterogeneous nodule 22 x 8mm in size with irregular borders and spicules or lateral prolongations. An infiltrating ductal carcinoma was diagnosed.

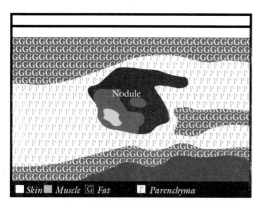

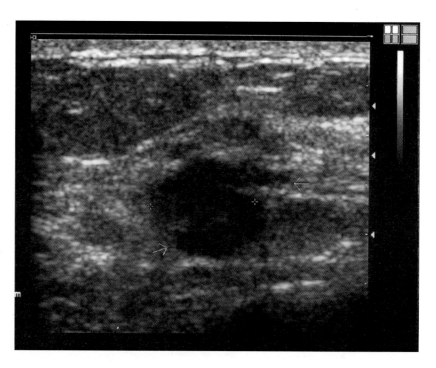

Figure 5.61 Image of a solid, heterogeneous nodule with irregular borders and a spicule-shaped prolongation. It was diagnosed as a ductal carcinoma.

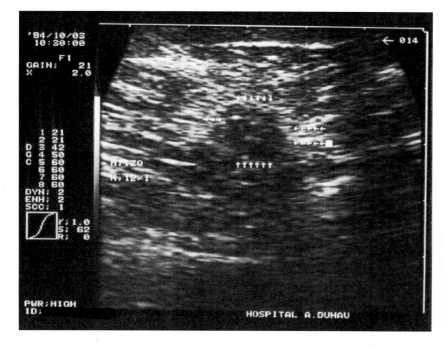

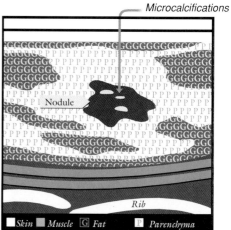

Figure 5.62 Image of a solid nodule with poorly defined borders and microcalcifications. An infiltrating ductal carcinoma was diagnosed.

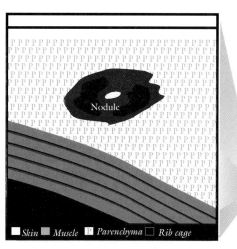

Figure 5.63 Image of a solid, heterogeneous nodule with interior microcalcifications and an irregularity on one border. It was diagnosed as a ductal carcinoma.

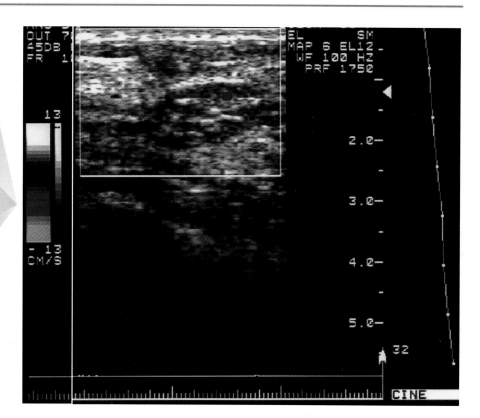

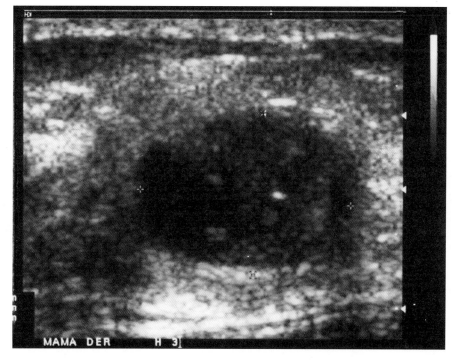

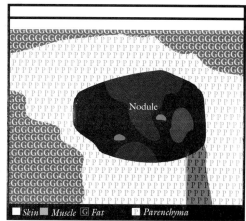

Figure 5.64 Image of a solid, heterogeneous nodule with partial posterior sonic attenuation. A ductal carcinoma was diagnosed.

Up to 40% of malignant tumors produce a posterior enhancement, or display a normal posterior border (however, this sign it is more commonly found in benign tumors, occurring in up to 95% of these).

A normal posterior border is most often seen in the following carcinomas: papillary, medullary, mucinous, and ductal infiltrating with necrobiotic areas.

There is often a capsule or crown of greater echogenicity around malignant tumors, which is caused by either tumoral infiltration of tissues, or a desmoplastic reaction in surrounding tissues.

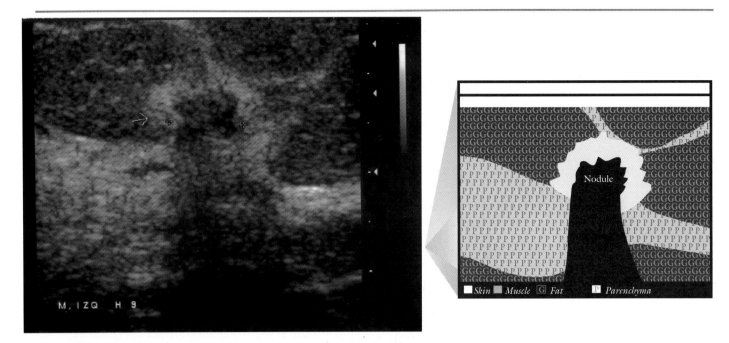

Figure 5.65 Image of a nodule with a hyperechogenic crown in a patient diagnosed with inflammatory carcinoma.

Tumors which are non-palpable or smaller than 1 cm have special characteristics. Sonographically these tumors may be similar to large tumors, but the combination of all the criteria of malignancy is found in these tumors only 30-40% of the time.

Only 20% of these tumors have (at least) one sign indicating malignancy, while 50% may appear benign or present as "borderline" cases.

The most frequent signs of these tumors (50-60%) are:
- **Irregular borders.**
- **Heterogeneous internal structure.**

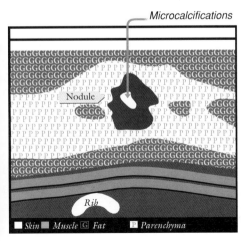

Figure 5.66 Image of a solid nodule 7mm in diameter with heterogeneous interior echoes due to microcalcifications. An infiltrating ductal carcinoma was diagnosed.

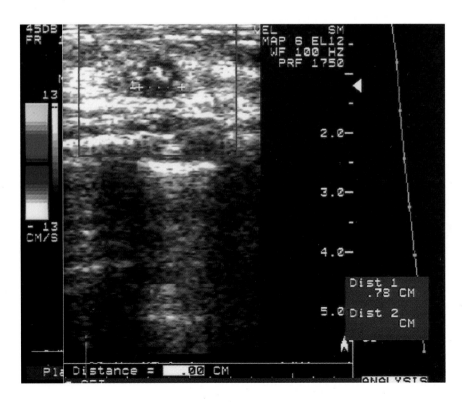

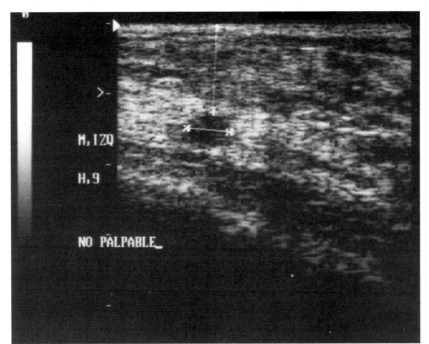

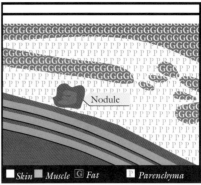

Figure 5.67 Image of a solid, non-palpable nodule 5mm in diameter located at a depth of 12mm with somewhat irregular borders. It was diagnosed by puncture as a carcinoma.

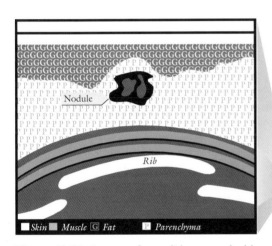

Figure 5.68 Image of a solid, non-palpable nodule 4mm in diameter. A ductal carcinoma was diagnosed.

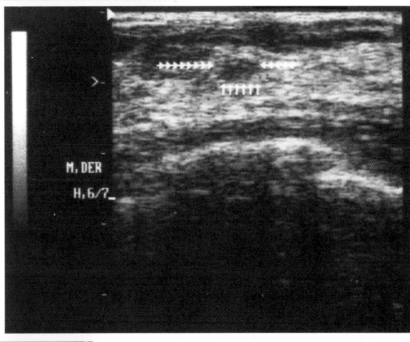

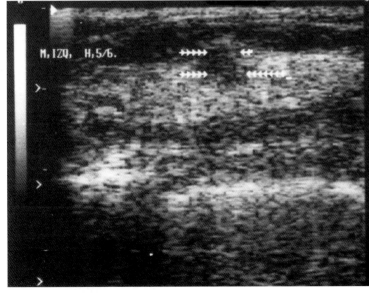

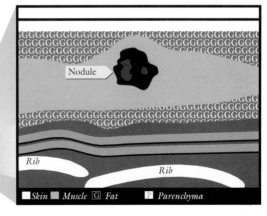

Figure 5.69 Image of a solid, non-palpable nodule 5 x 6mm in size with slightly ill-defined borders. Infiltrating ductal carcinoma.

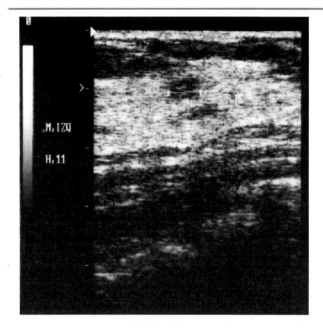

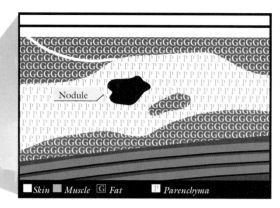

Figure 5.70 Image of a solid, non-palpable nodule 5mm in size with heterogeneous echoes. It was diagnosed by puncture and biopsy as a carcinoma.

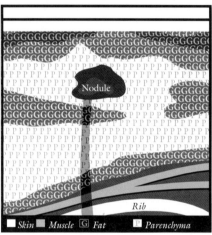

Figure 5.71 Image of a solid, non-palpable nodule 4 x 5mm in size which displays posterior sonic attenuation in one sector. Biopsy showed an infiltrating ductal carcinoma.

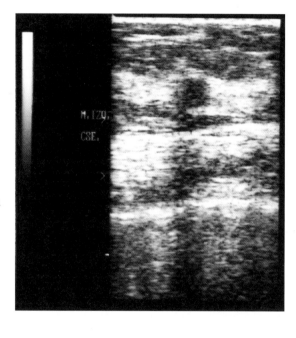

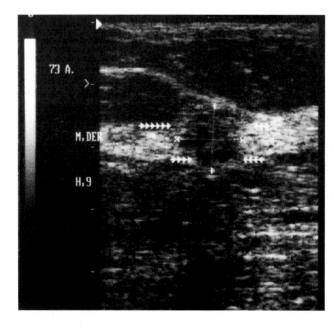

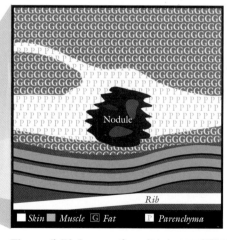

Figure 5.72 Image of a solid, hypoechoic nodule 10 x 11mm in size in a 73 year-old patient. It was diagnosed as neoplasia.

Sonic attenuation is encountered in 13% of tumors which are non-palpable or smaller than 1 cm; 30% of them have their greatest diameter perpendicular to the skin.

These tumors can be difficult to diagnose due to their similarity to benign tumors. For this reason it is wise to employ an ultrasound-guided (US-guided) puncture to aid in diagnosis.

As a general rule, the first step in the diagnosis of a nodule is to ensure that it has none of the following signs of malignancy:

- **Decrease in echogenicity.**
- **Microlobulation.**
- **Angled border.**
- **Sharply pointed calcifications.**
- **Spiculations.**
- **Partial or total sonic attenuation.**
- **Intraductal extension.**

Ultrasound in the Clinical Diagnosis of In Situ Carcinoma

Numerous sites of ductal *in situ* carcinoma may be found, and they may manifest themselves in the following ways:

- **Ductal papillary mass.**
- **Calcifications.**
- **Solid nodule with microcalcifications; signs of branching or intraductal expansion.**

When this type of carcinoma displays microcalcifications, they typically have the following characteristics:

- **Small and highly echogenic.**
- **Generally do not present sonic attenuation.**
- **May be located within a dilated duct, within a nodule, or in papillary lesions.**

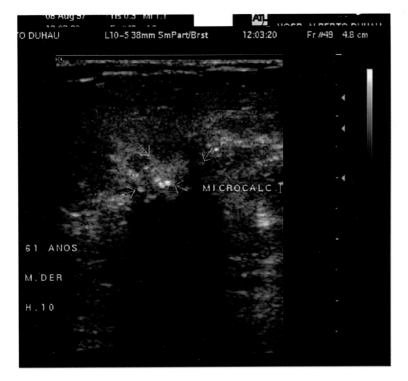

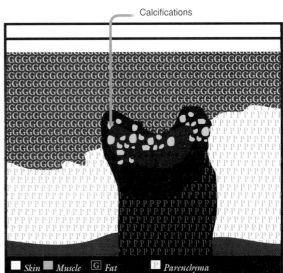

Figure 5.73 Image of a nodule located in the upper-outer quadrant of the right breast of a 61 year-old patient. There is considerable tissue destruction and sonic attenuation as well as spicules and multiple calcifications. It was diagnosed as a ductal carcinoma (histological degree II, nuclear degree III, and mitotic index III) with areas of comedocarcinoma but no signs of skin infiltration or axillary metastasis.

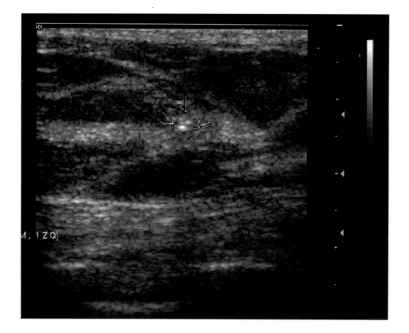

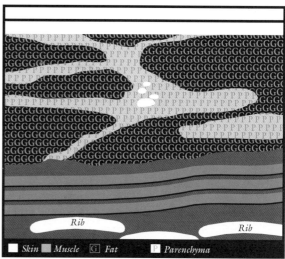

Skin ■ Muscle G Fat P Parenchyma

Figure 5.74 Image of a cluster of microcalcifications without sonic attenuation within thinned glandular parenchyma. Diagnosed as an *in situ* lobular carcinomas with a cribbed pattern and areas of chronic comedomastitis.

Synchronous bilateral carcinoma has an incidence rate of 3.6%, which makes it necessary to perform an exhaustive preliminary bilateral mammographic analysis. The analysis should then be correlated with an ultrasound examination.

The most common sonographic signs of invasion by carcinoma are:

- **Spiculations.**
- **Echogenic crown.**
- **Angled margins.**
- **Sonic attenuation.**

60% to 80% of invasive carcinomas may also display an *in situ* carcinoma. These are most often found in the peripheral sector of the nodule.

An ultrasound evaluation should be performed in cases where intraductal extension is suspected. The most commonly encountered sonographic signs of intraductal extension are:

- **Ducts which appear both solid and dilated.**
- **Microlobulations with hyperechogenicity.**
- **Branching.**

The surgical plan for a circumscribed carcinoma is very different of that for a carcinoma with possible intraductal extension. Therefore, the importance of adequate equipment and utmost thoroughness in the search for signs of intraductal extensions cannot be overstated.

One of the primary causes of recurrence in cancers is the insufficient excision of cancerous tissue. In the case of a circumscribed carcinoma conservative surgical therapy may be sufficient, but in cases of possible ductal extension the resection must be ample enough to remove the affected tissues.

Breast Carcinoma without a Demonstrable Nodule

According to an article published by Tohno et al. there have been cases of carcinomas which did not present a visible nodule and were diagnosed by ultrasound because of the following signs:

- **Intraductal dilatation.**
- **Contents of the ducts.**
- **Increase in the width of the parenchyma in a specific sector.**
- **Distortion and decrease of echogenicity in any sector.**
- **Strong echoes concentrated in one area.**

It must be emphasized that individually, these signs are not cause for suspicion, however; if a number of them are encountered, one should perform both clinical and mammographical examinations, and if necessary perform a US-guided puncture.

References

- Bruneton J, Caramella E, Michel H, *et al.*: Axillary lymph node metastasis in breast cancer: Preoperative detection with US. *Radiology* 1986; 158:325-326.
- Tate JJ, Archer L, Guyer P, Royle G, Taylor I: Ultrasound detection of axillary lymph node metastases in breast cancer. *Eur J Sug Oncol*, 1989; 15:139-141, de Freitas R, Costa MV, Schneider SV, *et al.*: Accuracy of ultrasound and clinical examination in the diagnosis of axillary lymph node metastases in breast cancer. *Eur J Surg Oncol*, 1991; 17:240-244.
- Pamilo M, Soiva M, Lavast EM: Real time ultrasound, axillary mammography and clinical examination in the detection of axillary lymph node metastases in breast cancer patients. *J Ultrasound Med*, 1989; 8:115-120.
- Wallis M, Walsh MT, Lee JR: A review of false negative mammography in a symptomatic population. *Clin Radiol*, 1991; 44:13-15.
- Mann BD, Guilano AE, Bassett LW, *et al.*: Delayed diagnosis of breast cancer as a result of normal mammograms. Arch Surg 1983; 118:23-24.
- Ma L, Fishell E, Wright B, *et al.*: Case-control study of factors associated with failure to detect breast cancer by mammography. *J Natl Cancer Inst* 84; 1992:781-785.
- Donegan WL: Evaluation of a palpable breast mass. *N Engl J Med*, 1992; 327:937-942.
- Harper PA, Kelly-Fry E, Noe JS, Bies RJ, Jackson VP: Ultrasound in the evaluation of solid breast masses. *Radiology*, 1983; 146:731-736.
- Jackson VP: Sonography of malignant breast disease. *Semin Ultrasound CT MR*, 1989; 10:119-131.
- Cole-Beuglet C, Soriano RZ, Kurtz B, *et al.*: Ultrasound analysis of 104 primary breast carcinomas classified according to histopatohological type. *Radiology*, 1983; 147:191-196.
- Cole-Beuglet C, Soreano R, Pasto M, *et al.*: Solid breast mass lesions: can ultrasound diferentiate benign and malignant? In: Jellins J, Kobayashi T, eds.: *Ultrasonic examination of the breast.* New York, NY. Wiley, 1983; 45-55.
- Adler DD: Breast masses: differential diagnosis. In: Feig SA, ed.: *ARRS categorical course Syllabus on breast imaging.* Reston, Va. American Roentgen Ray Society, 1988; 231-240.
- Kasumi F: Can microcalcitications located within breast carcinomas be detected by ultrasound imaging? *Ultrasound Med Biol*, 1988; 14: (supp. I); 175-182.
- Sickles EA: Sonographic detectability of breast calcifications. *Proc. SPIE*, 1983; 419:51-52.
- Wadden NAT: Breast ultrasound. In: Wilson SR, Charboneau JW, Leopold GR, eds.: *ARRS ultrasound categorical course syllabus.* Reston, Va. American Roentgen Ray Society, 1993; 199-204.
- Calderon C, Vikomerson D, Mezrich R, Etzold FK, Kingsley B, Haskin M: Differences in the attenuation of ultrasound by normal, benign and malignant breast tissues. *JCU*, 1976; 4:249-254.
- Egan RL, Egan KL: Detection of breast carcinomas classified according to histologic type. *Radiology*, 1983; 147:191-196.
- Hall FM, Storelld JM, Silverstone DZ, *et al.*: Non-palpable breast lesions: recommendations for biopsy based on suspicion of carcinoma at mammography. *Radiology*, 1988; 167: 353-358.
- Marquet KL, Funk A, Fendel H, Handt S: The echo-dense edge and hyper-reflective spikes: sensitive criteria for malignant proccsses in breast ultrasound. *Geburtshilfe Frauendheilkd*, 1993; 53:20-23.
- Teubner J: The echogenic border: an important diagnostic criterion in sonographic tumor diagnosis of the breast. In: Gill RW, Dadd MJ, eds.: *World Federation of Ultrasound in Medicine and Biology*, 1985. Oxford, England, Pergammon, 1985; 342.
- Nishimura S, Matsusue S, Loizumi S, *et al.*: Size of breast cancer on ultrasonography, cut surface of resected specimen, and palpation. *Ultrasound Med Biol* ,1988; 14 (supp. I); 139-144.
- Gordon PB, Gilks, B: Sonographic appearance of normal intramammary lymph nodes. *J Ultrasound Med*, 1988; 7:545-548.
- Cole-Beuglet C, Soriano RZ, Kurtz, AB, Goldberg, BB: Ultrasound analysis of 104 primary breast carcinomas classified according to histopathologic type. *Radiology*, 1983; 147:191-196.
- Ueno E, Thono Y, Hirano *et al.*: Ultrasound diagnosis of breast cancer. *J Med Imaging* 1986; 6:178-188.
- Buell P: Changing incidence of breast cancer in Japanese-American women. *J Nat Cancer Inst*, 197; 51:1479-1483.
- Trapido EJ: Age at first birth, parity and breast cancer risk. *Cancer* 1983; 51:946-948.
- Anderson DE, Badzioch MD: Risk of familial breast cancer. *Cancer* 1985; 56:383-387.
- Anderson DE: Breast cancer in families. *Cancer* 1977; 40:1855-1860.
- Meyer JE, Amin E, Lindfords KK, *et al.*: Medurally carcinoma of the breast: mammographic and US appearance. *Radiology*, 1989; 170:79-82.
- Kasumi F, Fukami A, Kuno K, Kajitani T: Characteristic echographic features of circumscribed cancer. *Ultrasound Med Biol*, 1982; 8:369-375.
- Cole-Beuglet C; Sonographic manifestation of malignant breast disease. Semin Ultrasound 1982; 3:51-57.

Diffuse Pathology of the Breast

M. E. Lanfranchi

Introduction

Ultrasound can be used to identify lesions before they become palpable or symptomatic, especially in young women and women with dense breasts. When ultrasound technology was introduced it was primarily used to differentiate small nodules from cysts in the breast. However, advances in ultrasound technology have made it possible to detect non-palpable nodules and lesions in the early stages of development.

Logically, the first step in the treatment of diffuse pathologies is detection, followed by differentiation, and finally diagnosis.

The breast undergoes three stages of development:
1) **Initial Stage**: Organization of histological components for later functional development.
2) **Functional Stage**: Breast is capable of responding to specific biological needs.
3) **Involutional Stage**: Breast loses its functional capacity.

All three stages are subject to hormonal stimulation, and microscopic zones of both cellular proliferation and involution are often observed. The breast is dynamic and subject to different modifications in each stage.

The predominance of any of these processes is referred to as dysplasia. Dysplasia is defined as "an alteration, disorder, aberration, disturbance, or persistant acquired anomaly of the mammary gland (including both ductal and connective components) presumably due to a hormonal imbalance (of estrogens, progesterone, or prolactin) which acts on the gland and can result in cyclic mastalgia and nodularity". It is a non-fatal, benign disorder, neither invasive nor metastasic.

In certain cases dysplasia may lead to fibrocystic disease (FCD), a pathology which:
- **Appears only in women who have a menstrual cycle.**
- **Varies according to the menstrual cycle.**
- **Involves a number of cycles or stages which constitute one process.**

FCD affects the entire parenchyma of the mammary gland, with differerent degrees of intensity in each zone. It is a common pathology, affecting between 30% and 50% of caucasian women according to some studies. It can be treated with hormones or other types of medical treatment.

Pathological Stages of FCD

There are three recognized developmental stages:

1) **Deficient stage:** Mastodynia (most common between 18 and 30 years of age).

Cyclic mastodynia is caused by a histological deficit in lobule formation during puberty. It may produce diffuse fibrosis, a paucity of blood vessels, and absent or apparently atrophied lobules; cysts do not form.

2) **Prolific or Hyperplastic Stage:** Adenosis (most common between 25 and 40 years of age).

Adenosis is characterized by uneven growth and development of the solid component of the gland and the canaliculi. There is solid proliferation of the papillae and zones of cavitation (in the form of cysts). The most commonly encountered forms of adenosis are: sclerosing adenosis, epitheliosis, papillary adenosis, cystic adenosis and involutive adenosis.

3) **Involutional Stage:** Sclerocystic mastopathy or Reclus' disease (most common between 35 and 55 years of age).

This stage is characterized by lobular atrophy without evidence of proliferation. The degree of physiological involution, not the degree of atrophy itself, constitutes dysplasia. The dysplasic elements of these pathologies generally manifest themselves as either single or multiple macrocysts.

Pain is frequent; it is generally bilateral and diffuse, but can also be predominant in one area. If the pain is cyclic, it will be exaggerated in the pre-menstrual period.

Pain is intense in the case of mastodynia, moderate in the case of adenosis, and slight or absent in the case of cysts.

Presence of Nodules

The development of nodules is progresive, and conforms to the three stages discussed above. In the deficient stage (mastodinia) there is, in addition to pain, irregularity in the gland, primarily in the upper-outer quadrant.

In the hyperplastic stage (adenosis) the presence of nodules is more pronounced and there is diffuse tumescence, primarily in the upper-inner quadrant. In some cases breasts affected by this disease are described as being similar to a bag of beans or marbles, and in others there is one dominant nodule.

There are two symptoms which indicate the involutional stage (sclerocystic mastopathy or Reclus' disease):

a) **Irregular induration, caused by fibrosis of the stroma.**
b) **Cysts, which appear as well-defined nodules.**

As in FCD's, the cyst develops in the mammary tissues. Pain is only experienced if the cyst forms rapidly.

FCD may be generalized (40%), or it may affect three-fourths of the breast (40%). When this disease is localized in one area it usually manifests itself as a well-defined cyst. However, if there are numerous cysts within the breast their borders will not be well-defined.

The ultrasound image may simultaneously display localized dysplastic areas and single or multiple cystic areas. FCD may manifest itself in a number of forms, each with a distinct ultrasound image.

Classification of Ultrasound Images of FCD

- **Diffuse pattern.**
- **Multiple bilateral foci.**
- **Localized pattern (focus).**
- **Single or multiple cysts.**
- **Complex pattern.**

The **diffuse pattern** usually appears in young women with dense breasts. There is generally a diffuse increase of echogenicity (often in the external sectors of the breast)

which corresponds to the area where pain is experienced. There is an increase in the thickness of the parenchyma, rather than the presence of nodules.

Multiple bilateral foci are often palpable and create echogenic alterations. In some cases there may be an increase in echogenicity, and in others, depending on the extent of fibrosis, the image may appear pseudonodular with both heterogeneous echostructure and a solid pattern.

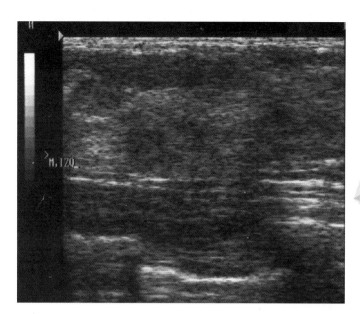

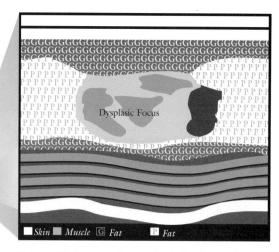

Figure 6.1 Image of a poorly defined nodular area at the level of the upper-outer quadrant which corresponds to a palpable induration. It was diagnosed as an area of dysplasic mastopathy.

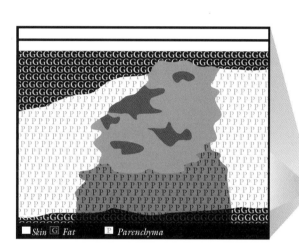

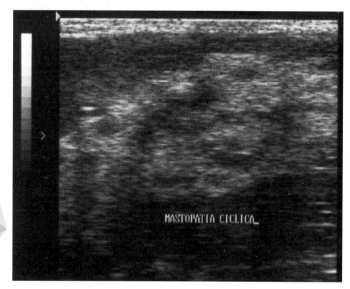

Figure 6.2 Heterogeneous pseudonodular areas in a patient with antecedents of mastopathy.

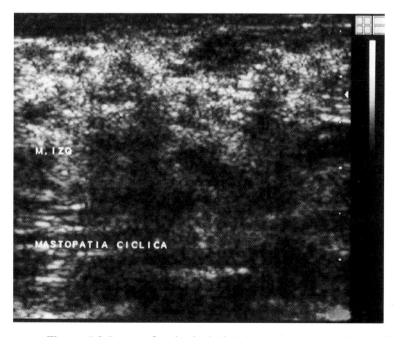

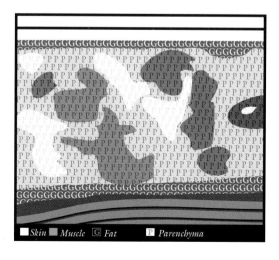

Figure 6.3 Image of a gland which is heterogeneous but lacks defined nodules. A diffuse dysplasic mastopathy was diagnosed.

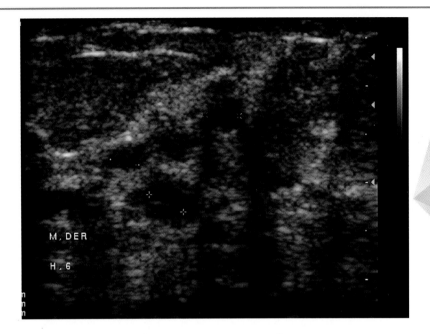

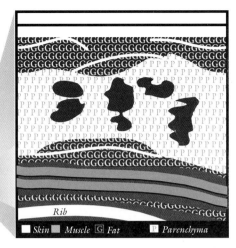

Figure 6.4 Multiple cysts of various sizes in a 34 year-old patient with FCD. Cysts appear as multiple hypoechoic areas, and cause alterations in the glandular echostructure.

When the pattern is localized it is referred to as a **dysplasic focus**; it is generally nodular with partially defined borders, which makes it difficult to distinguish from the gland itself in some areas. For this reason an ultrasound-guided (US-guided) cytological or histological puncture may be necessary in order to perform a differential diagnosis.

Single or multiple cystic images are generally seen in breasts with heterogeneous parenchyma, with areas of increased echogenicity. Breasts affected by fibrosis also appear heterogeneous, and generally display palpable cysts. Often these patients have been diagnosed with dysplasia a number of years earlier; the cysts themselves are either anechoic with well-defined borders and posterior enhancement, or appear as solid nodules with fine interior echoes due to the accumulation of secretions. In these cases a puncture is necessary for diagnosis.

The **complex image** is produced by a combination of the types discussed above, in various proportions and locations within the breast.

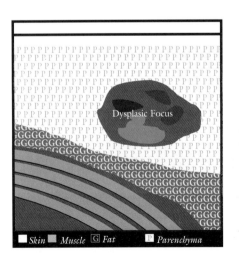

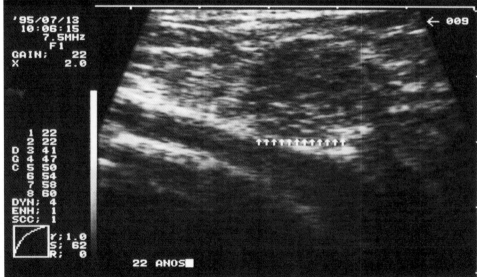

Figure 6.5 Image of a diffuse area of lower echogenicity due to dysplasic mastopathy in a 22 year-old patient complaining of a painful, palpable induration. It disappeared completely after treatment.

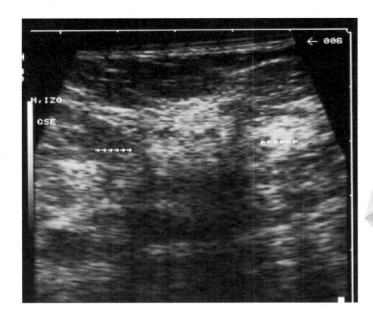

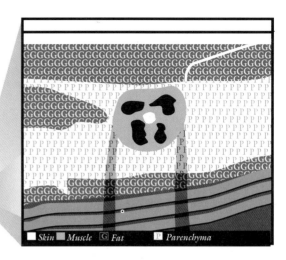

Figure 6.6 Image of an area of increased echogenicity which corresponds to a dysplasic focus. Similar images were observed in other sectors of the breast.

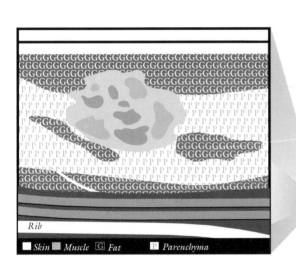

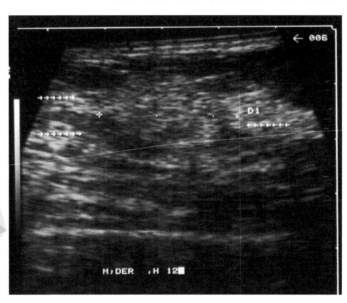

Figure 6.7 Image of a dysplasic, pseudonodular area displaying increased echogenicity.

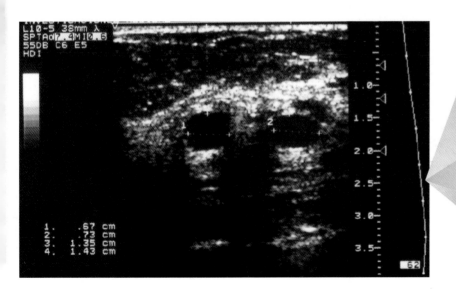

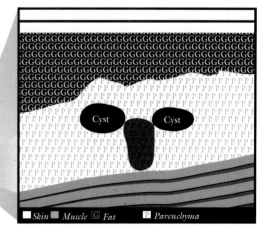

Figure 6.8 Image displaying an alteration in the echogenicity of the parenchyma between two simple cysts in a patient diagnosed with FCD.

Benign Lesions Associated with FCD

Cysts are the most frequent lesions associated with FCD, occurring in 20% to 22% of all cases; half of these are solitary cysts.

Cysts located within areas of localized dysplasia occur in 18% of all cases. Other pathologies, such as fibroadenoma, phyllodes tumor, or papillary tumor occur in a total of 5% of all cases.

Dysplasia and Cancer

According to J.V. Uriburu et al., 12.2% of all dysplasias involve cancers. In another study a group of 500 radiologically-diagnosed cancers were examined, 16.8% of which were encountered in cases of dysplasia.

Although these numbers indicate that the incidence of cancers related to dysplasias is low, it is important to take diagnostic measures to ensure that cancer is not present.

Diabetic Mastopathy

This is a rare disease which affects diabetic patients who are insulin-dependent. These patients display an alteration of the echogenicity of the parenchyma. In some cases there is considerable sonic attenuation, which makes it necessary to perform a differential diagnosis with other mass-occupying pathologies. Histological studies of these sectors display only fibrosis.

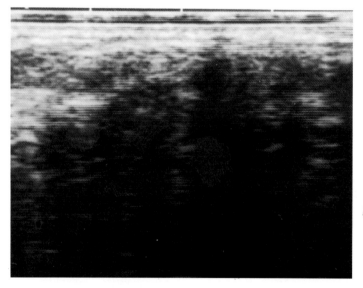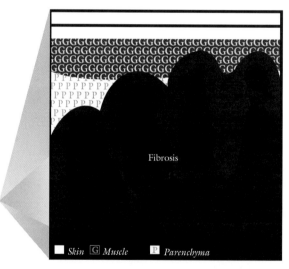

Figure 6.9 Image of an area with a considerable decrease in echogenicity in a patient with mammary fibrosis due to diabetic mastopathy.

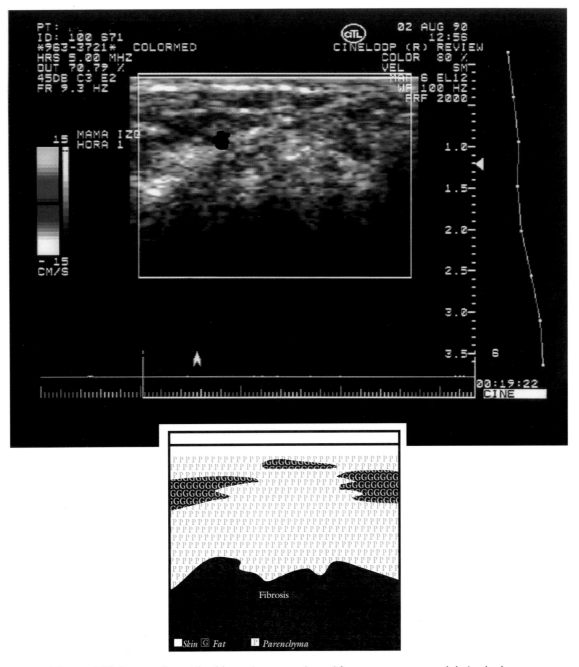

Figure 6.10 Image of considerable sonic attenuation without an apparent nodule in the lower half of the parenchyma of a patient with diabetic mastopathy. Mammary fibrosis was diagnosed.

References

- Uriburu JV y col. *La mama, tratado de mastología.* Tomo I, vol I. Parte general y procedimientos diagnósticos. Buenos Aires, 1996.
- Gruhn JG, Staren ED, Wolter J: *Breast cancer. The Evolution of Concepts.* Ed. Field & Wood. Inc. Pennsilvania.
- Harris JR, Hellman S, Henderson IC, Kinne DW: *Breast Diseases,* 2nd. ed. J. B. Lippincott Co. Philadelphia, 1991.
- Uriburu JV: *Las displasias mamarias en la obra de Astley Cooper. Cir Panamer,* 2: 385, 1959.
- Hughes LE, Mansel RE, Webster, DJT: *Benign Disorders and diseases of the breast.* Ed. Bailliere Tindal. London, 1989.
- Frantz AG: The breasts. En : Williams, R.H.: *Textbook of Endocrinology.* W.B. Saunders Co. Philadelphia, 1981.

7

Ultrasound Examination of the Lactiferous Ducts

M. E. Lanfranchi

The lactiferous ducts appear in ultrasound images as tubular, radial hypoechoic structures which converge near the nipple. The diameter of each main duct increases below the areola in a dilation known as the ampulla.

These ducts sometimes divide into two or three secondary or tertiary ducts wich run paralell to one another. When viewed from a perpendicular angle these ducts will appear to be stacked on top of one another; when viewed from above they will seem to be one duct.

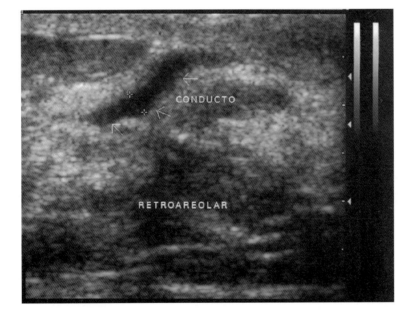

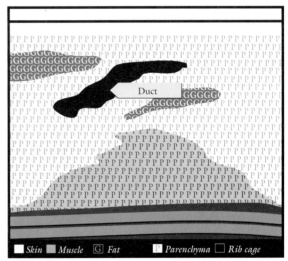

| Skin | Muscle | G Fat | P Parenchyma | Rib cage |

Figure 7.1 Image of a lactiferous duct close to the areola which lies in an oblique angle to the skin. It has a normal diameter of 2mm.

It must be kept in mind that the nipple has only between 6 to 8 lactiferous pores, and that the ducts join in groups of 2 or 3 in order to form the main collectors and arrive at the nipple.

This anatomical arrangement explains the difficulties encountered in attempting to penetrate the ducts in a scan. Ultrasound examinations of this area must be performed with great care, taking into consideration the ductal topography.

The technique employed for the examination of this area is different from that used in other areas. To examine the ducts, radial sections of the breast should be scanned, in order to find the longitudinal axis of the ducts. Then, if a pathology is detected, the area should be examined in transverse sections.

Breast Ultrasound

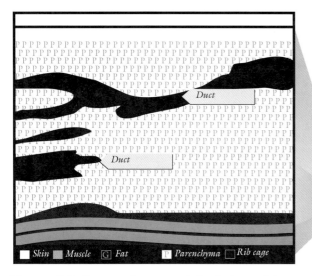

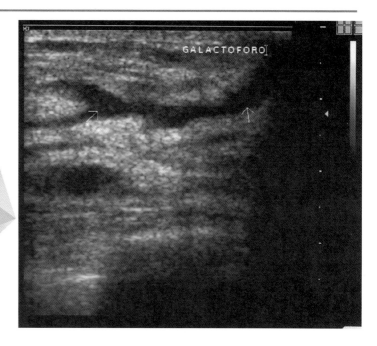

Figure 7.2 Image of a normal-sized duct with a bifurcation and a curved, horizontal trajectory.

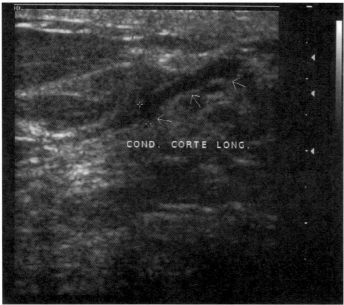

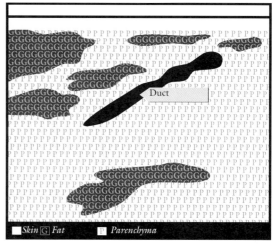

Figure 7.3 Image of a duct taken at a perpendicular angle which displays a slightly irregular (but still within normal limits) posterior wall.

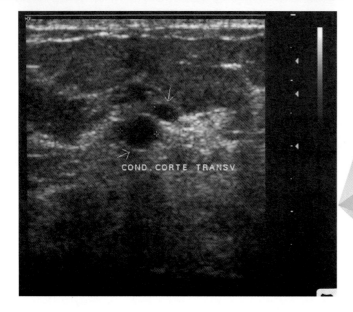

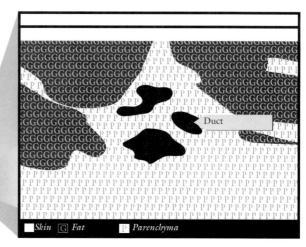

Figure 7.4 Transverse section of a number of ducts; viewed from this angle they can be mistaken for cysts.

In cases in which the patient experiences discharge from the nipple, it is the best to induce the discharge in a systematic manner in order to determine which sector is affected. Once determined, a detailed examination of the sector should be made.

In order to obtain sufficient contrast to permit evaluation of the walls and contents of the ducts (the ducts are hypoechoic in relation to the rest of the parenchyma), one should emphasize the use of the power gain variations in both the grey scale and the close field. Good image definition and a wide focalization of the close field are also necessary. Thus, proper equipment is a must for ductal examinations; transducers of at least 7.5 MHz, and in some cases 10 MHz, should be used.

Ultrasound examinations of the ducts are performed for three main reasons:

1) **Secretion or discharge from the nipple.**
2) **Doubtful or non-conclusive mammography.**
3) **The ducts may be examined while performing an ultrasound for other reasons.**

Nipple discharge is defined as "the abnormal secretion of a liquid from the nipple" which occurs spontaneously or due to manipulation of the nipple area.

One should keep in mind that nipple discharge and secretion are symptoms which often accompany cancers. According to various investigators, its incidence rate may be 3% (Haagensen), 7.4% (Leis), or 8.7% (Uriburu).

The accumulation of liquid may be due to pathologies either within or outside of the walls of the ducts.

Pathologies located outside the ductal walls may be:
- **Tumoral invasion** of the ducts, after an inflammatory reaction and subsequent destruction of the wall.
- **Inflammation** and edema of the gland, or purulent exudation which later flows into the lumen of the duct.

Pathologies located within the walls may be:
- **Epithelial proliferation**, in dysplastic papillomatosis, benign papillary tumors, or ductal cancers.
- **Infection** of the ductal wall.
- **Necrosis** of the tissues.
- **Lesions** of the vessels (eg. intraductal hemorrhagic granuloma).

The discharge may have the following characteristics:
- **Milky secretion** due to causes (other than childbirth) located outside the breast (hyperprolactinemia, tumor of the C.N.S., pharmaceuticals, etc).
- **Bloody secretion**, marked by the presence of red blood cells.
- **Non-bloody** secretion or discharge; serous, purulent, with a yellowish-green hue.

According to a study by Uriburu et al., hemorrhagic secretions are the least frequent (27.2%), yet the most dangerous; non-hemorrhagic secretions make up the remaining 72.8%. Table 7.1 below gives the percentages of the various pathologies constituting 506 cases of nipple secretion.

Pathology	Percentage
Fibrocystic disease (FCD)	53%
Papillary tumor	15.4%
Ductal ectasia	11.2%
Cancer	7.5%
Galactophoritis	4.7%
Hemorrhagic intraductal granuloma	1.2%
Dysplastic papillomatosis	0.3%

Table 7.1

Approximately 10% of all cases of FCD involve secretion from the nipple, and each of the three stages of the disease display a distinct type of secretion (although, in some cases all three stages may co-exist in the same gland). Secretions accompanying mastodynia are composed of cells from the ductal walls; they can be bilateral and affect various pores. However, secretions are uncommon.

In cases of adenosis secretion is concentrated in one or more pores; it is generally serous, or in the case of hyperplasia and papillary formations in the ducts, bloody-serous.

In the fibrocystic stage secretion is concentrated in one or more pores; is generally yellowish-green and has a creamy consistency. It is caused by papillary proliferations of the epithelium and inflammatory processes. FCD is the most common benign breast disease; it involves the formation of cavities or cysts which triggers a fibrotic reaction in the surrounding connective tissue. These cysts are due to a localized dilation in the ductal system and can cause pain, nodulation, cystic masses, or may pass undetected in clinical examinations because of their small size.

Cysts can be classified in four ways using ultrasound: by size (microcysts when smaller than 5 mm); by appearance (simple or complex cyst); by the type of fibrocystic pathology; or according to their original location (ductal, lobular, ductal-lobular).

Ductal cysts develop in the lumen of one or more ducts. Generally, there are multiple cysts; they are often found in the same stage of development and follow the trajectory of the duct. They may, in some cases, accompany ductal hyperplasia or irregularities in the ductal wall.

Lobular cysts are often multiple and are localized in bunches near the periphery of the lobe. These cysts are generally found in different sizes and stages of development.

Ductal-lobular cysts may be multiple; they have irregular borders and augmented echogenicity in their walls due to fibrosis of the surrounding tissues.

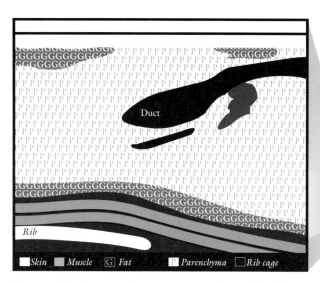

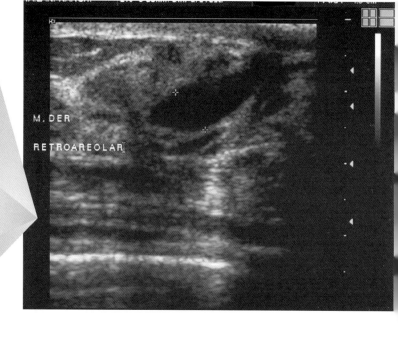

Figure 7.5 Image of retromammary-located lactiferous ducts, the largest of which is 6mm in diameter in a patient with FCD.

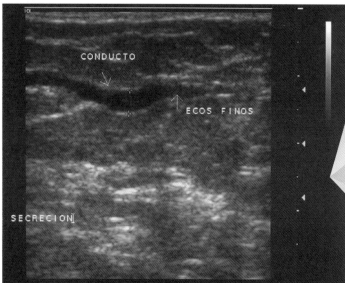

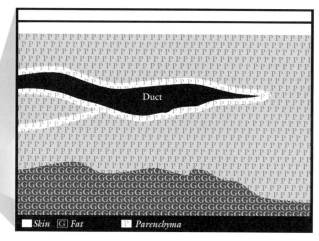

Figure 7.6 Image of an undilated duct 3mm in diameter in a patient complaining of a serous secretion from the nipple. The duct has fine echoes in one area and is located in the center of an area affected by FCD.

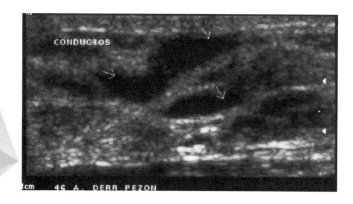

Figure 7.7 Image of ducts between 2 and 4mm in diameter in a patient complaining of a yellowish serous secretion from the nipple. Small echoes appear in an area of FCD.

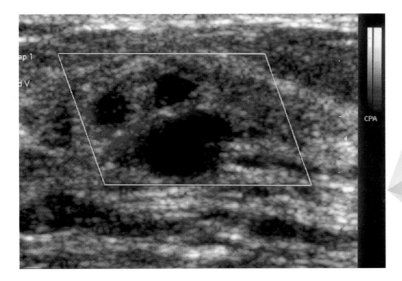

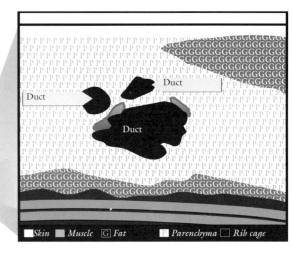

Figure 7.8 Image of an area of dysplasic mastopathy displaying multiple dilated ducts which have a cyst-like appearance. The signal is weak and peripheral using Power.

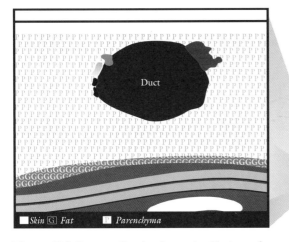

Figure 7.9 Image of a simple cystic dilation of a duct. The use of Color Doppler shows the direction of flow into two sectors.

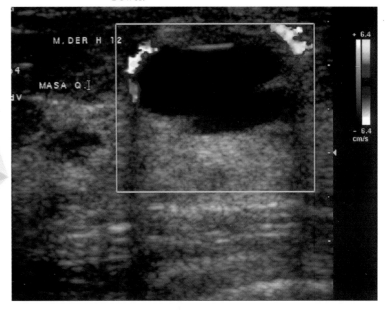

Ductal-lobular cysts sometimes appear as hypoechoic pools of liquid, or with fine echoes adjacent to their walls due to cellular detritus.

In such cases three areas should be examined by ultrasound-guided (US-guided) puncture in the following order:

    1) The tissues surrounding the cyst.
    2) The area of fine echoes adjacent to the walls.
    3) The remaining areas of the cyst.

The examination should be performed in this order and before obtaining a sample of the liquid filling the cyst, in order to avoid collapsing the area of interest. A US-guided puncture is prudent because, although it is rare that a cancer develops within a ductal-lobular cyst, it can occur.

This type of adenosis is described in a study by Urban as a non-encapsulated lobular hyperplasia which displays a proliferation of both ducts and acini. In the case of pure adenosis the number and size of both ducts and acini is augmented; if followed by fibrotic reaction, the pathology is referred to as adenosclerosis.

According to Leis et al., adenosis is a hyperplasia of the lobular epithelium. The ultrasound image is that of a group of dilated lobules, the extremities of which contain fibrotic tissue with a round or triangular shape and a liquid center.

Ductal ectasia, defined as a dilation of the ducts, may be found in 3% of benign mastopathies, and approximately 50% of these cases involve secretion (1 of every 8 cases of secretion will be non-hematic).

This pathology is most often found in perimenopausal women; it can be either unilateral or bilateral, discharge a yellowish, greenish, or brown liquid, and is at times accompanied by umbilication of the nipple. Secretion is caused by desquamation of epithelial cells accompanied by inflammation or infection.

Dilation cannot normally be detected by clinical or mammographical examinations. Occasionally a soft mass is palpable beneath the areola, and liquid discharge from the nipple may be observed.

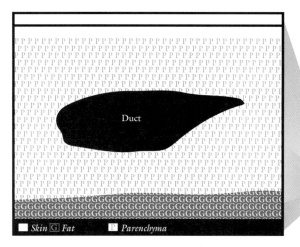

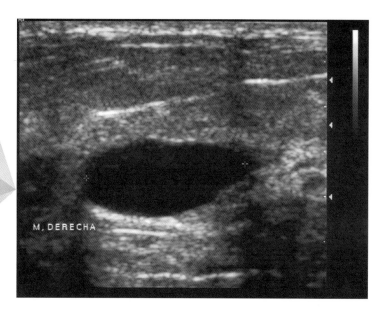

Figure 7.10 Image of an 18mm segmental dilated duct which resembles a cyst.

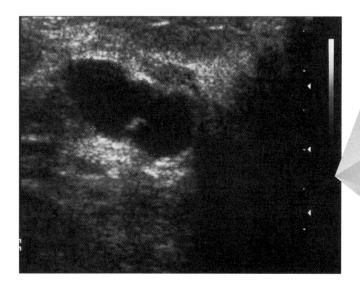

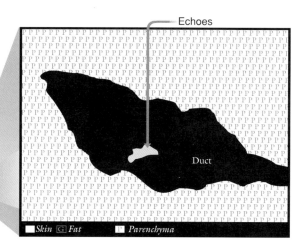

Figure 7.11 Image of a lacunar segmental dilated duct with an accumulation of fine echoes in one area due to cell detritus.

Ductal ectasia begins as a dilation of the retroareolar portion of the ducts, which may extend towards the lobules (although this is rare).

The liquid within the ducts may be clear, or it may produce fine echoes due to the presence of desquamative cells or red blood cells.

The borders or walls of the duct may become irregular over time, and the surrounding tissue may display fibrotic reaction.

Aspirating a duct will cause its collapse, and the type of liquid obtained varies according to the complications involved with the pathology and the stage at which it was discovered.

Ductal ectasia involves a moderate risk of cancer, so it should be closely and carefully monitored.

Papillomas and papillomatosis are the fourth most common diseases of the breast and consist of papillary proliferations of the ductal endothelium which partially fill and may distend the duct.

In general this is a non-palpable pathology and its proliferations are no more than a few millimeters in size. It may appear in cysts, dutal ectasias, and carcinomas. Three types of images may be observed:

- **A small mass, single or multiple, inside a duct or a ductal ectasia.**
- **A pedunculated image inside the lumen.**
- **Vegetations inside a cystic dilation or a retroareolar duct.**

When there is evidence of multiple masses, microcystic pathologies or hyperplasia an US-guided biopsy or a surgical excision may be neccessary.

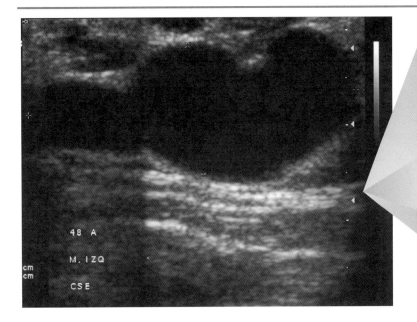

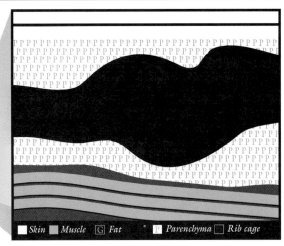

Figure 7.12 Image of a segmental dilated duct 35 x 13mm in size in a 48 year-old patient complaining of a palpable nodule. A puncture produced a serous liquid and collapsed the duct.

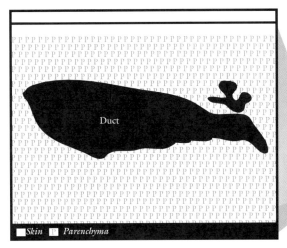

Figure 7.13 Image of a segmental dilated duct displaying enhancement of the duct wall due to an older process.

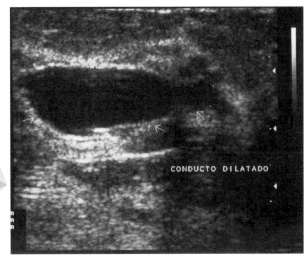

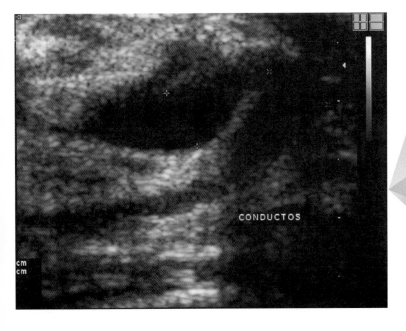

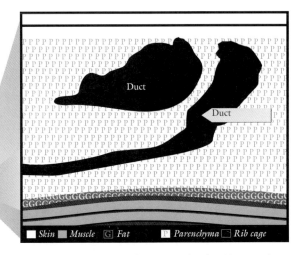

Figure 7.14 Image of retroareolar lactiferous ducts with a maximum diameter of 5mm; all are asymptomatic.

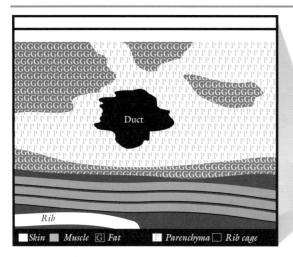

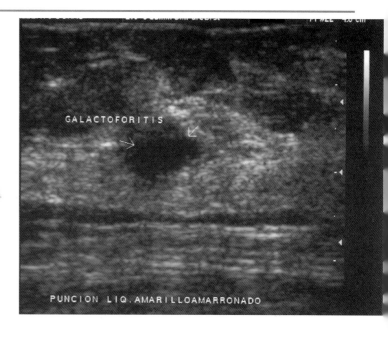

Figure 7.15 Transverse section of a lactiferous duct with somewhat irregular borders. Punture produced a yellowish-brown liquid indicative of galactophoritis.

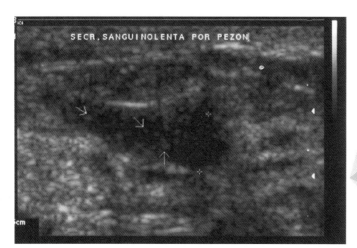

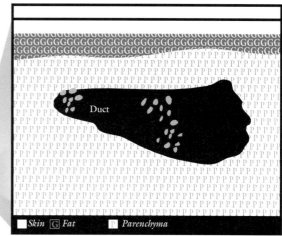

Figure 7.16 Image of a benign pathology in a patient complaining of a bloody secretion from the nipple. Fine echoes within the duct are caused by red blood cells.

Echoes

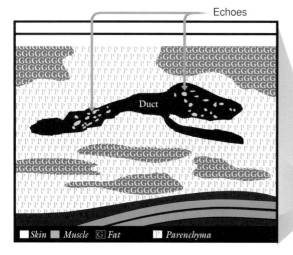

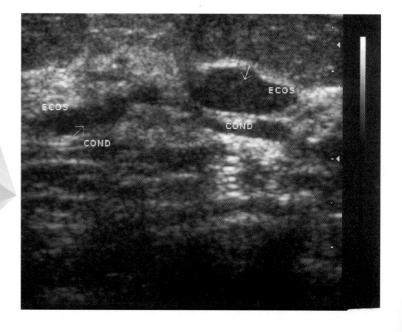

Figure 7.17 Image of ducts with irregular borders, fine interior echoes and a fibrotic reaction in the neighboring tissues. Galactophoritis.

140

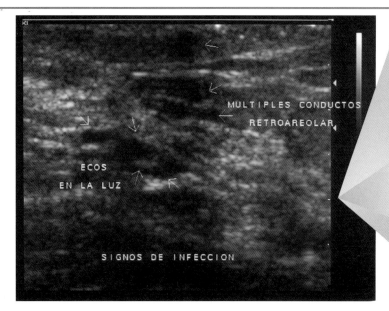

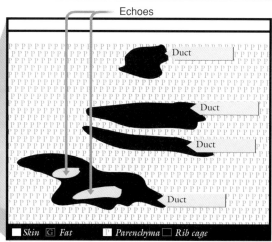

Figure 7.18 Image of multiple ducts of normal size, some with fine interior echoes, in a patient with signs of an inflammatory process and infection near the areola. She was successfully treated with antibiotics.

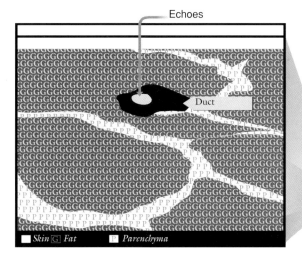

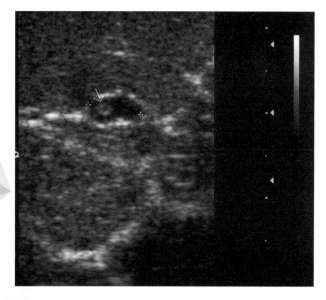

Figure 7.19 Image of a 6mm duct with an interior papilloma which appears as a small mass.

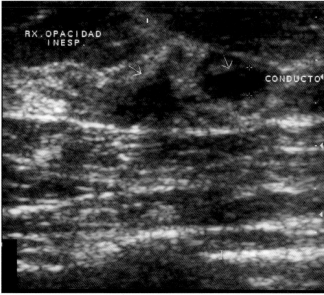

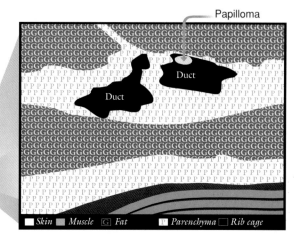

Figure 7.20 Transverse section of two ducts, one which contains a benign papilloma, in a patient with unspecific mammary opacity.

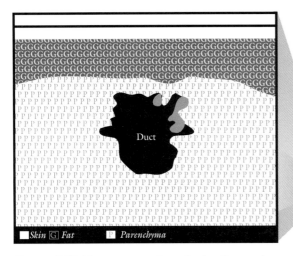

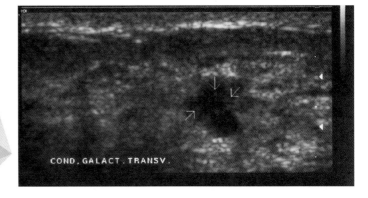

Figure 7.21 Transverse section of a lactiferous duct with a benign papilloma.

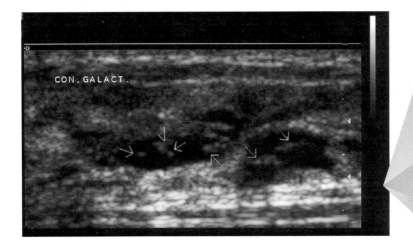

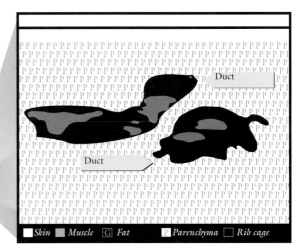

Figure 7.22 Image of lactiferous ducts which display multiple vegetations due to a papilloma.

Any cancer affecting the breast can be accompanied by secretion from the nipple, depending on the anatomical and histological characteristics of the tumor. In scirrhous cancers, for example, this symptom has never been observed, while it is frequent in ductal neoplasias. Geschikter has found that 36% of secretions from the nipple are due to ductal cancer, and in 10% of ductal cancers secretion is the first symptom.

On the other hand, any histological type of infiltrating cancer, when it invades the wall of a duct, may produce bloody secretions.

An article published by Teboul divides breast cancers affecting the ducts into three types:

- **Lobular (10%).**
- **Focal ductal-lobular (10%) and focal ductal (60%).**
- **Diffuse (20%).**

In its initial stages the lobular type presents multiple independent foci along the length of the duct.

Although bloody secretions may be caused by papillary cancer (papillary tumor types III or IV) they are more commonly caused by benign tumors (type I and II).

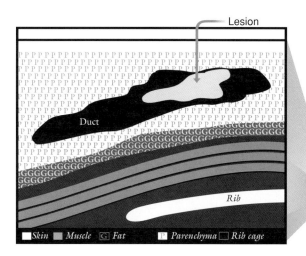

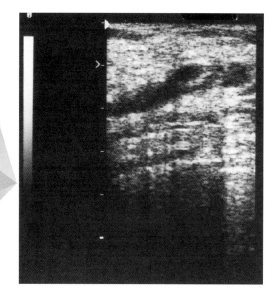

Figure 7.23 Image of a lactiferous duct which displays an interior hyperechogenic mass in a patient complaining of a bloody secretion from the nipple. A carcinoma was diagnosed.

Type I, as seen in figure 7.24, is non-palpable and only a few millimeters in size. It is located inside a main duct and does not affect the entire wall.

Type II, as seen in figure 7.25, is often retroareolar, occupies the entire lumen of the dilated duct, and has papillary-type cells.

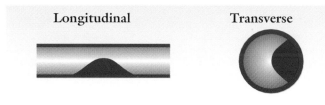

Figure 7.24

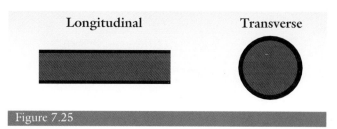

Figure 7.25

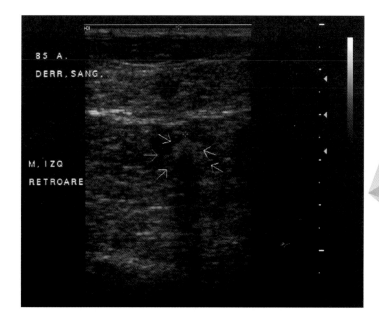

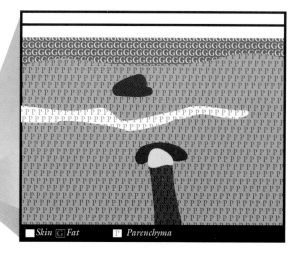

Figure 7.26 Image of retroareolar duct occupied by an echogenic mass at a depth of 23mm in an 85 year-old patient complaining of a spontaneous bloody discharge from the nipple. The mass was diagnosed as a malignant papillary tumor.

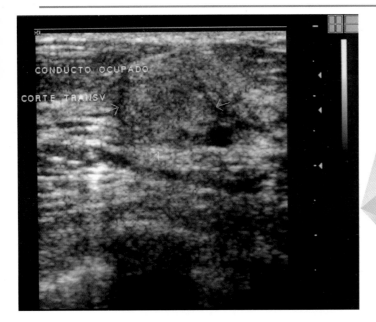

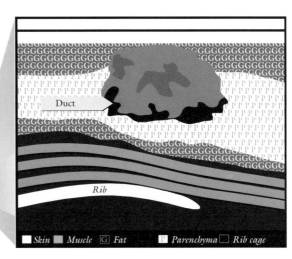

Figure 7.27 Transverse section of a lactiferous duct completely occupied by a solid heterogeneous mass diagnosed as a papillary tumor.

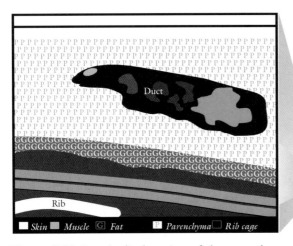

Figure 7.28 Longitudinal section of the same duct from Figure 7.27.

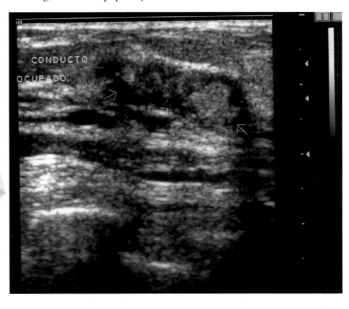

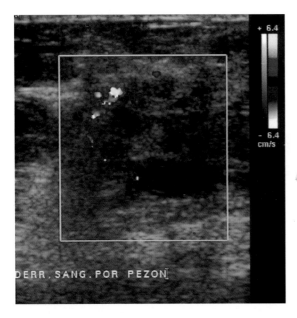

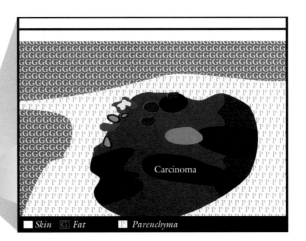

Figure 7.29 Image of several heterogeneous ducts in a 62 year-old patient with abundant and continuous bloody secretion from the nipple. It was diagnosed as a ductal carcinoma which affects the walls of several ducts.

Tumors type I and II are referred to as interductal papilloma or dentritic adenoma.

Secretion may present in both palpable and non-palpable tumors. One should differentiate between the palpation of a tumor and that of duct dilated by secretion (a dilated duct, once evacuated, should be less palpable).

When a duct contains secretion, its walls become irritated and inflammed, which may lead to chronic or erosive galactophoritis (erosive galactophoritis tends to produce a bloody secretion).

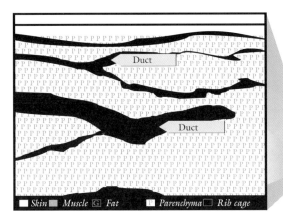

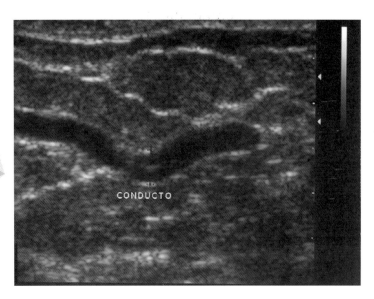

Figure 7.30 Image of a duct 3mm in diameter with regular and defined borders. Galactophoritis.

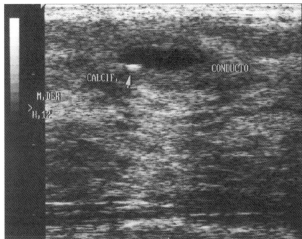

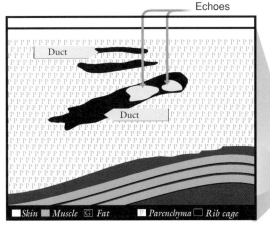

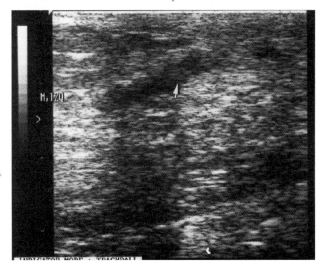

Figure 7.31 Image of a duct with discrete focal ectasia and a small calcification on one wall due to an inflammatory disease.

Figure 7.32 Image of a lactiferous duct displaying numerous interior echoes in a 67 year-old patient suffering from bloody secretion from the nipple. A benign papillary lesion was diagnosed.

145

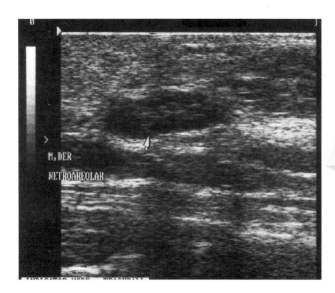

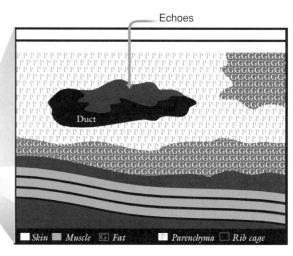

Figure 7.33 Image of a lactiferous duct displaying fine interior echoes. Diagnosis by cytological puncture was galactophoritis.

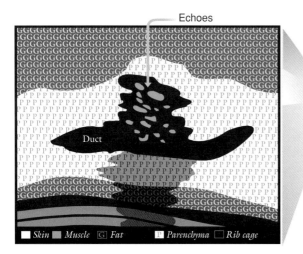

Figure 7.34 Image of ducts with partially defined borders and fine echoes in several areas. Cytological puncture confirmed galactophoritis.

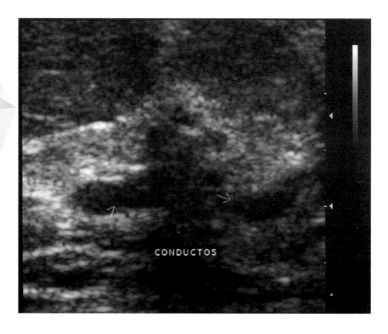

Hemorrhagic intraductal granuloma is a rare lesion caused by inflammation of the ductal wall. It produces a small mass within the dilated duct and may cause blood in the lumen.

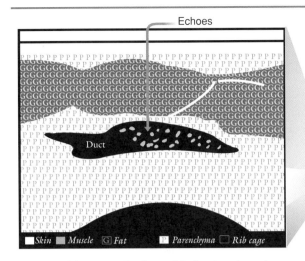

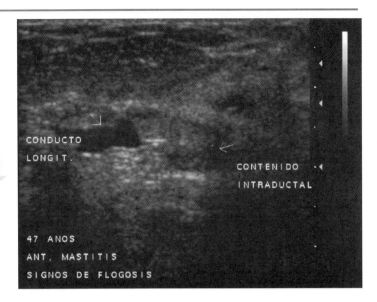

Figure 7.35 Image of a duct with fine interior echoes in a patient with a prior mastitis and showing signs of inflammation. Interior echoes were caused by purulent material.

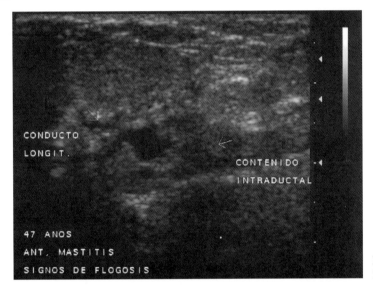

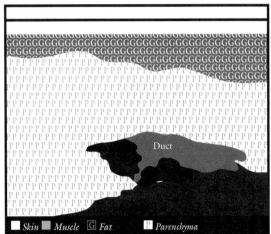

Figure 7.36 Another sector of the ducts from Figure 7.35.

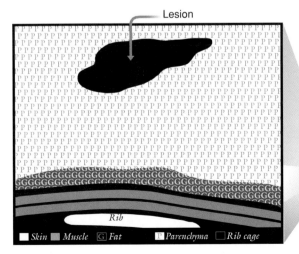

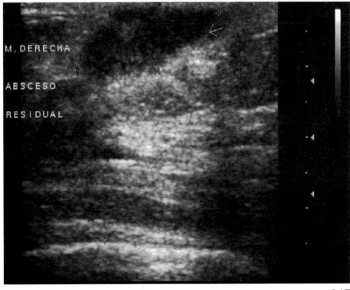

Figure 7.37 Image of a hypoechoic area near the nipple in a patient with a prior mastitis and complaining of a white discharge from the nipple. Punture confirmed a residual abscess.

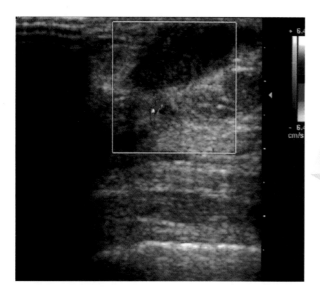

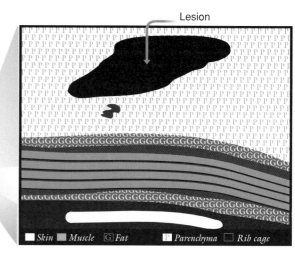

Figure 7.38 Color Doppler image of the pathology in Figure 7.37 showing a weak signal in a peripheral area indicating an inflammatory process in the surrounding tissues.

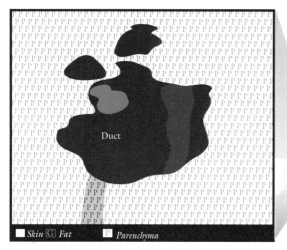

Figure 7.39 Image of a dilated and irregular duct displaying heterogeneous echoes in a patient with a history of breast pain and tumefaction. She was treated successfully with antibiotics.

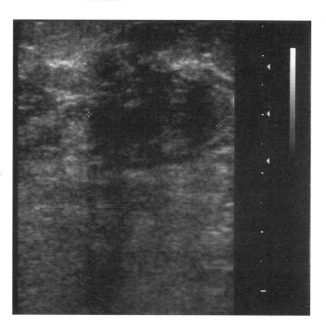

To summarize, in the case of ductal pathologies one should examine:

- **The ductal wall.**
- **The contents of the duct.**

The findings may be (Fig. 7.40):

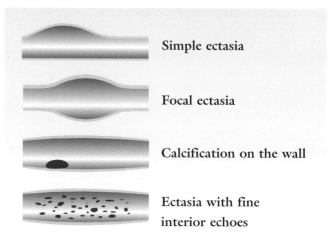

Simple ectasia

Focal ectasia

Calcification on the wall

Ectasia with fine interior echoes

Figure 7.40

The mass inside the duct may occupy:

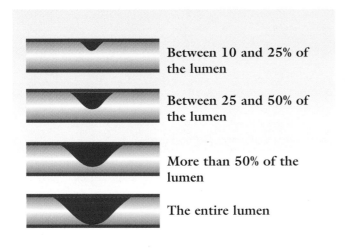

Between 10 and 25% of the lumen

Between 25 and 50% of the lumen

More than 50% of the lumen

The entire lumen

Figure 7.41

In general terms there are two possiblities:
- **Secretion without a tumor.**
- **Secretion with a tumor.**

Of course, one must bear in mind that secretion is only a symptom, and investigate its cause. The secretion of pus or pus and blood, for example, is a symptom which can accompany both benign and malignant pathologies.

If there is a tumor in addition to secretion, the tumor should be investigated promptly in order to reach a diagnosis and establish an appropriate treatment.

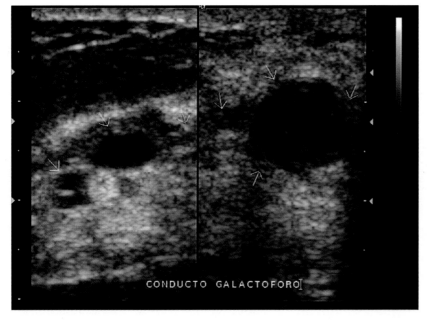

CONDUCTO GALACTOFORO

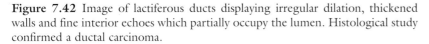

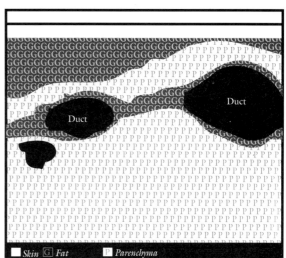

Skin G Fat P Parenchyma

Figure 7.42 Image of lactiferous ducts displaying irregular dilation, thickened walls and fine interior echoes which partially occupy the lumen. Histological study confirmed a ductal carcinoma.

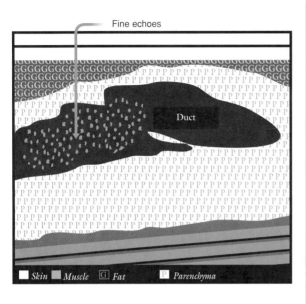

Fine echoes

Skin Muscle G Fat P Parenchyma

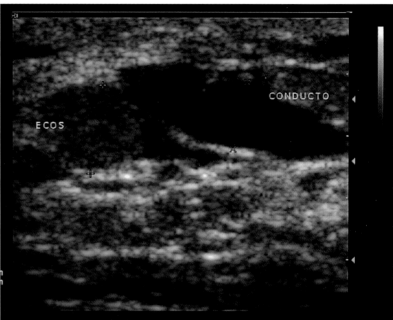

CONDUCTO

ECOS

Figs. 7.43, 7.44 Images of dilated ducts of variable and irregular diameter displaying fine interior echoes in one area, in a patient complaining of a bloody secretion from the nipple. A chronic galactophoritis was diagnosed by puncture.

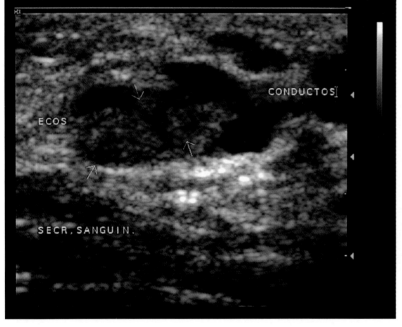

CONDUCTOS

ECOS

SECR. SANGUIN.

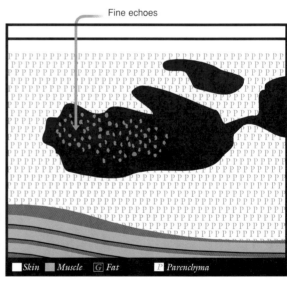

Fine echoes

Skin Muscle G Fat P Parenchyma

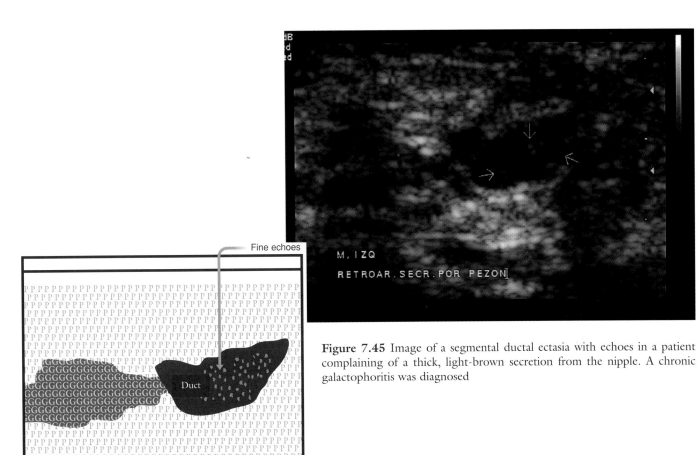

Figure 7.45 Image of a segmental ductal ectasia with echoes in a patient complaining of a thick, light-brown secretion from the nipple. A chronic galactophoritis was diagnosed

References

- Kamio, T., Kameoka, S., et al. (1993). Ductal Echography. International breast Ultrasound School. Procceding of the 8th. International Congress on the ultrasonics examination of the breast 1-4 July 1993. Heidelberg. p. 52.
- Teboul, M. (1993). Ductal echography splits the rol of mammography Proceedings of the 8th International Congress on the Ultrasound examination of the breast. 1-4 July 1993. Abstract p. 28.
- King, E. B., Goodson, W. H. (1991). Pérdidas y secrecciones por pezón Editorial Saunders. Philadelphia.
- Leis, H. P. et al. (1985). Nipple discharge: significans and treatment. Breast 11 (2): 6.
- Leis, H. P. (1989). Management of Nipple Discharge. World J. Surg. 13:736.
- Uriburu, J. V. y col. (1996). La mama. Tratado de Mastología, 1, p. 102-129.

Trauma and Infections

M. E. Lanfranchi

Introduction

Breast traumas are, by definition, painful and thus clinical examinations and mammographies are difficult for both the patient and the clinician. Ultrasound is the best examination method in these cases.

Blunt traumas, such as those caused by striking the steering wheel in a car accident, may cause the following lesions:

- **Contusion.**
- **Hematoma.**
- **Fat necrosis.**

If the trauma results in an open wound which compromises the skin and subcutaneous tissues, the following may result:

- **Tissue destruction.**

- **Hematoma.**

Any of these lesions may affect the skin, the subcutaneous tissue, and all or part of the gland depending on the severity of the trauma.

The most common clinical findings are:

- **Pain.**
- **Ecchymosis.**
- **Edema.**
- **Induration or nodule.**

Contusions generally result from mild traumas; in general ultrasound images display an alteration in the echogenicity of various layers, without evidence of blood extravasation.

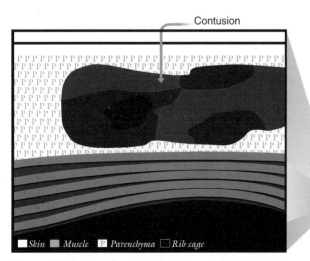

Figure 8.1 Image of a contusion in a patient who had undergone a trauma 15 days prior. The area of the contusion appears hypoechoic, heterogeneous, and displays partially defined borders.

☐ *Skin* ■ *Muscle* ᴾ *Parenchyma* ☐ *Rib cage*

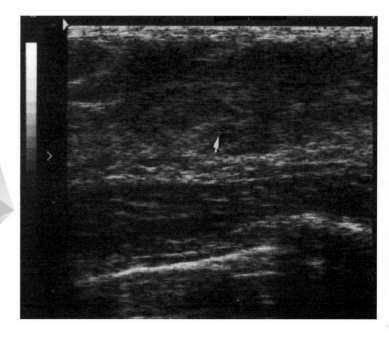

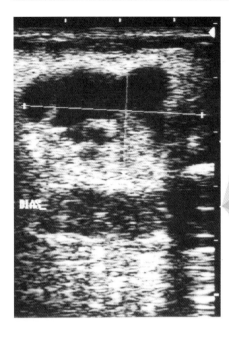

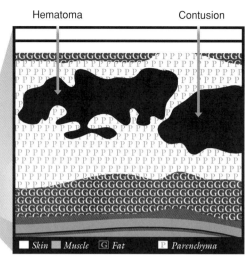

Figure 8.2 Image of a contusion in a 70 year-old patient who had undergone a trauma 12 days prior. There is an anechoic area with a liquid appearance due to hematoma and a hypoechoic area caused by the contusion.

Hematomas are caused by direct traumas (such as falls, blows, and knife or gunshot wounds) or surgical procedures. If blood vessels or capillaries are broken by the trauma, blood will collect in the tissues and remain in a liquid state for a short time before coagulating.

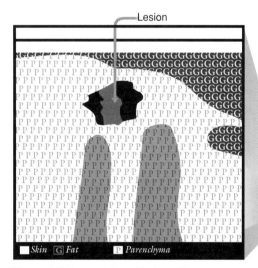

Figure 8.3 Image taken 21 days after a trauma displaying an area of liquid which indicates a hematoma.

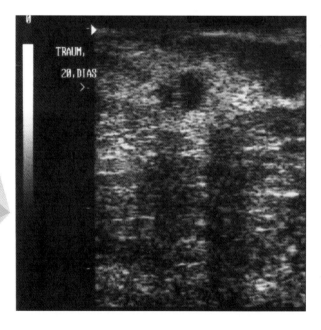

Once the blood begins to coagulate, the ultrasound image is more complex and heterogeneous due to the presence of liquid and pseudosolid areas (caused by the action of fibrin) which constitute an organized hematoma.

Regardless of whether they contain liquid or coagulated blood, hematomas have irregular borders which may be poorly defined in some sectors (normally in cases involving both contusions and hematoma).

Mammary contusions can cause fat necrosis, as soon as a month or as long as a year after the trauma.

Fat necrosis (sometimes referred to as lipophagic necrosis or citosteatonecrosis) manifests itself in either of the following forms during its initial period:

- **Oily cyst**; most often found after surgery.
- **Solid or complex nodule**; hypoechoic with poorly defined borders.

With time, areas of fat necrosis tend to calcify partially or completely, producing an image of very low echogenicity, with irregular and poorly-defined borders,

154

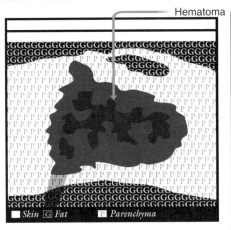

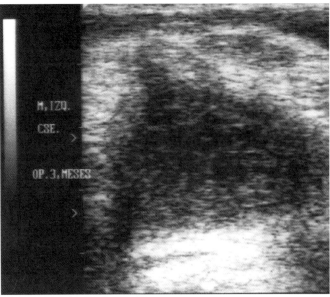

Figure 8.4 Image of a nodular mass with heterogeneous echoes and partially defined borders in a patient who had undergone breast surgery three months prior. An organized hematoma was diagnosed.

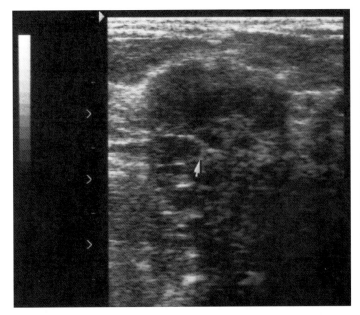

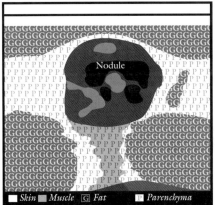

Figure 8.5 Image of a nodule with completely heterogeneous echostructure, irregular echoes, and partial attenuation in a patient who had undergone surgery 1 month prior. It was diagnosed as an organized hematoma.

and sonic attenuation. This makes it necessary to perform a differential diagnosis with a carcinoma (see Chapter 5).

Traumas in women with breast implants can damage the implants to various degrees, from small tears to complete ruptures, resulting in the contents of the implant entering the surrounding tissues.

Post-surgical granuloma is caused by surgical trauma; it appears as a solid image with partially defined borders and low echogenicity in all areas except the center (see Chapter 10).

Foreign bodies are occasionally visualized by ultrasound. Needles, for example, will appear as a continous line of increased echogenicity whose size corresponds to the needle's length and diameter.

Silicone injected into the breast appears sonographically as multiple cystic or liquid anechoic areas with irregular and possibly confluent borders (see Chapter 3, figure 3.9.).

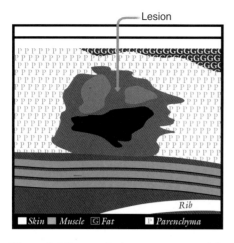

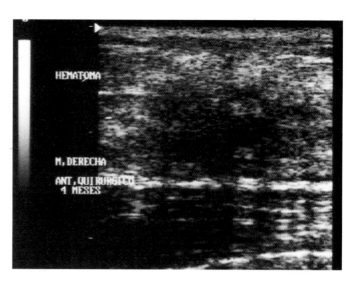

Figure 8.6 Image of a heterogeneous nodule with anechoic areas near the surgical scar of a patient who had undergone surgery three months prior. Organized hematoma.

Mastitis

Mastitis is a general term which refers to inflammations and infections of the breast. It may be acute, subacute, or chronic and can manifest itself in a number of different forms. Infections affecting the breast may originate in the gland itself or be caused by exterior factors. Nursing babies, for example, sometimes carry staphylococcus and spread infection to the breast. According to a study by Scholefield, mastitis caused by staphylococcus can affect up to 8.5% of nursing mothers.

Mastitis often presents with tumescence, localized warmth, fever, pain and general discomfort. 80% of mastitis cases occur in the first month post-partum, and 6% of the cases are bilateral. The infection may involve the gland (mastitis), the retroareolar region (galactophoritis), or the subcutaneous tissues.

Ultrasound images of acute mastitis generally display:
- **Edema and thickening of the skin.**
- **Alteration in the echogenicity of the tissues.**
- **Ductal ectasia.**
- **Increase in the volume of the gland.**
- **Dilation of lymph vessels parallel to the skin.**

Acute mastitis frequently leads to suppuration or abscess with poorly-defined and irregular borders, heterogeneous echoes in the interior and a decrease in echogenicity.

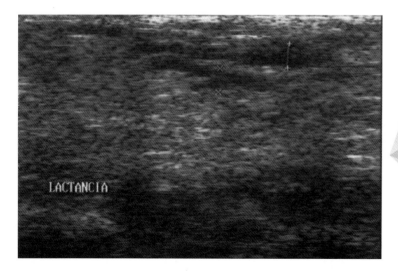

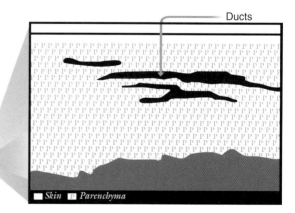

Figure 8.7 Image of a normal gland and galactophorous ducts in a lactating patient with signs of mastitis.

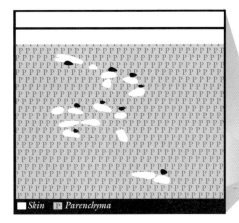

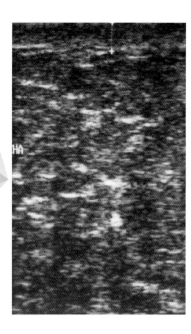

Figure 8.8 Image of a gland with mastitis displaying thickening of the skin and heterogeneous and hypoechoic parenchyma due to edema.

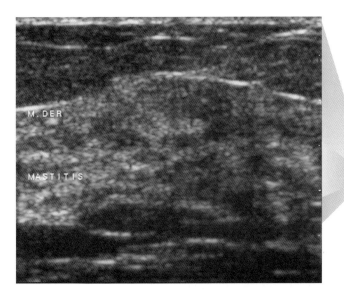

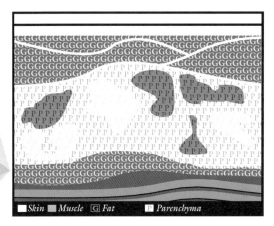

Figs. 8.9-8.11 Images of a gland with mastitis which has heterogeneous echostructure without nodules and without thickening of the skin.

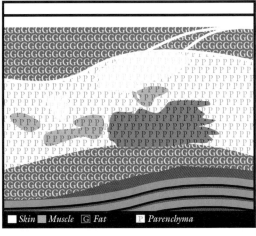

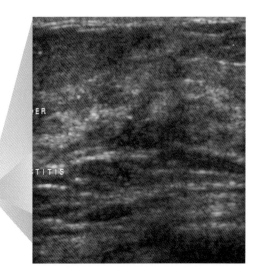

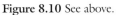

Figure 8.10 See above.

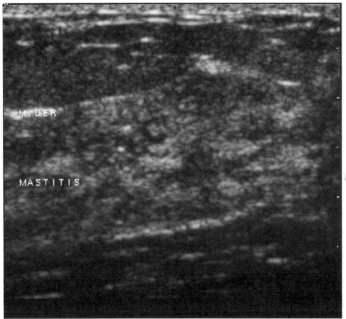

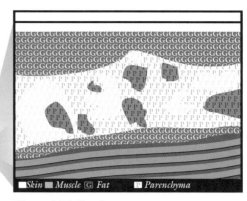

Figure 8.11 See above.

■Skin ■Muscle G Fat P Parenchyma

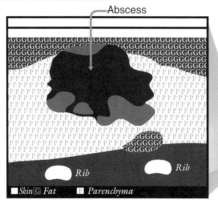

Abscess

■Skin G Fat P Parenchyma

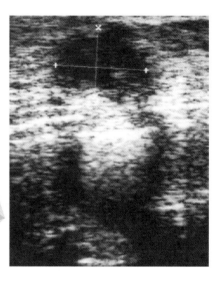

Figure 8.12 Image of an anechoic abscess displaying irregular borders and heterogeneous echoes on the wall.

According to research conducted by Geschikter, abscesses due to acute mastitis are rare, occurring in between 0.1 and 0.5% of cases of puerperal mastitis.

Acute mastitis, like other inflammatory processes, may evolve into granuloma or fibrosis, which in turn may lead to a chronic lesion or granulomatosis.

Chronic mastitis may be pyogenic, either evolving from acute mastitis, or having been chronic from the beginning.

Other types of chronic mastitis exist, but most are rare, caused by specific diseases such as tuberculosis, syphilis, actinomycosis, or parasitosis.

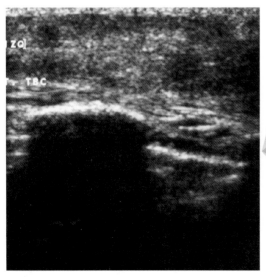

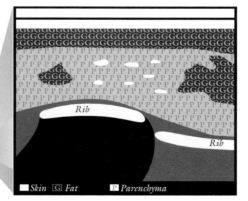

■Skin G Fat P Parenchyma

Figs. 8.13, 8.14 Images of a gland with areas of greater echogenicity and a few calcifications. Chronic mastitis caused by tuberculosis was diagnosed.

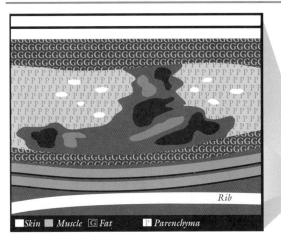

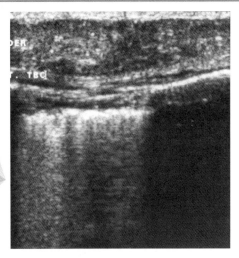

Figure 8.14 See above.

When the infection is located in the lactiferous ducts it may cause either galactophoritis or perigalactophoritis, which is frequently associated with ductal ectasia.

In these cases the ultrasound image displays tubular or cystic structures, with partially-defined borders and fine interior echoes.

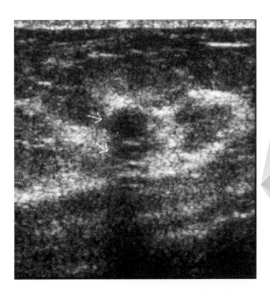

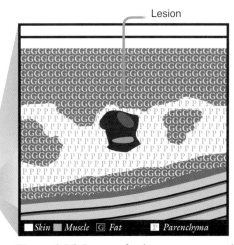

Figure 8.15 Image of a heterogeneous and hypoechoic mass diagnosed as galactophoritis.

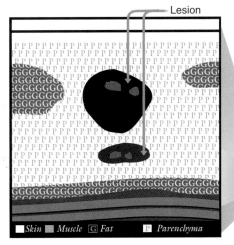

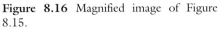

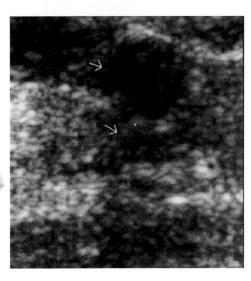

Figure 8.16 Magnified image of Figure 8.15.

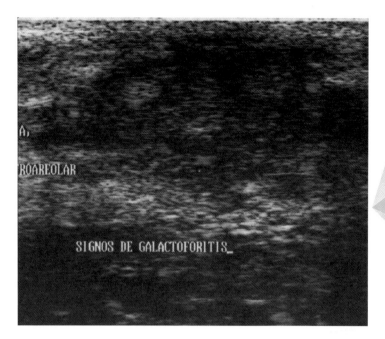

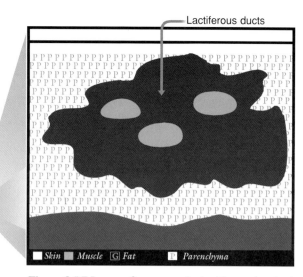

Figure 8.17 Image of a retroareolar lactiferous duct both hypoechoic and heterogeneous due to secretions in a patient complaining of discharge from the nipple. Galactophoritis.

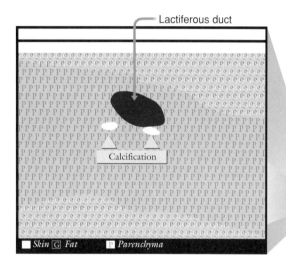

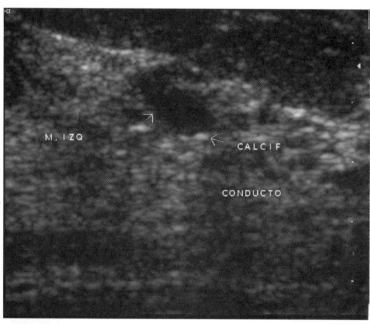

Figs. 8.18, 8.19 Sections of a lactiferous duct with small calcifications on its border. Galactophoritis.

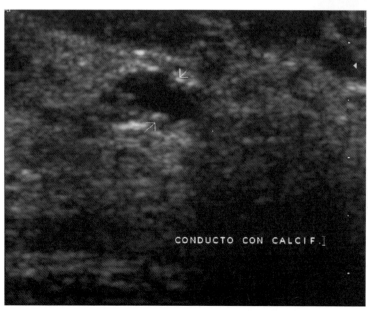

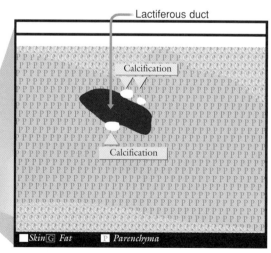

Figure 8.19 See above.

The skin of the breast contains hair follicles which are susceptible to furuncles and carbuncle. However, if these infections engage only the dermis they are subject to dermatological and clinical diagnosis.

If these infections appear in ultrasound images a differential diagnosis with other types of ductal pathologies should be considered (see Chapter 7).

Acute mastitis, for example, can be confused with the most serious of breast diseases, inflammatory carcinoma (see Chapter 5).

As stated previously, ultrasound can play an important role in cases of infectious pathologies, in diagnosis and evaluation of purulent collections, therapy, and subsequent follow-up.

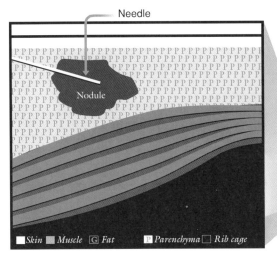

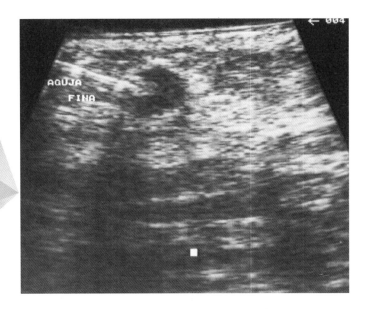

Figure 8.20 Image of a hypoechoic nodule 6 x 10mm in size in contact with the skin. The puncture needle can be seen in the upper left-hand corner. Galactophoritis.

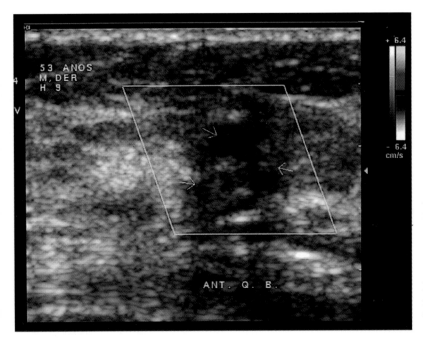

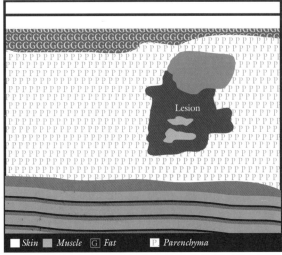

Figure 8.21 Image of a heterogeneous, hypoechoic area with irregular and partially defined borders in a 53 year-old patient with a scar due to previous surgery. Puncture confirmed it to be an area of fat necrosis.

References

- Rizzatto G, Chersevani R, Giuseppetti G M *et al.*: *Breast Ultrasound*. Bologna, Grasso, 1993.
- Bland KL: Inflammatory, Infectious and Metabolic Disorders of The Breast: In Bland KB, Copeland EM (eds): *The Breast*, Philadelphia, Saunders, 1991, pp. 87-112.
- Van Overhagen H, Zonderland HM, Lameris JS: Radiodiagnostic Aspects of Non-Puerperal Mastitis. *Fortschr Rontgenstr*, 1988; 149:294-297.
- Boisserie-Lacroix M, Lafitte JJ, Sirben C, *et al.*: Les lesions inflammatoires et infectieuses du sein. *J Radiol*, 1993; 74:157-163.
- Auquier MA, Baratte B, Grumbach Y: Conduit a tenir devant un sein inflammatoire. *Radiologie J CEPUR*, 1990; 10:49-56.
- Hayes R, Michell M, Nunnerley HB: Acute Inflamation of the Breast. The Role of Breast Ultrasound in Diagnosis and Management. *Clin Radiol*, 1991; 44:253-256.

9

Ultrasound of Mammary Prostheses

M. E. Lanfranchi

Introduction

The first report on the use of silicone breast prostheses was presented in 1963 by Cronin and Gerow and since that date many different techniques and materials have been used in this field. Reasearch and development in the area of breast prostheses has concentrated on achieving both chemical tolerance (to avoid rejection by the body) and mechanical tolerance (to increase comfort and avoid displacements).

Implant surgery is a common therapy for the following conditions:

 -**Congenital amastia.**
 -**Atrophy.**
 -**Mastectomy.**
 -**Mammary hypoplasia.**

Mammary hypoplasia is the most frequent condition for which implants are used (in Argentina alone for example there are approximately 200,000 patients who have ungergone implant surgery for this reason).

Implants consist of silicone rubber bags which contain silicone gel, saline solution, or in some cases hydrogel.

In 1992 the Food and Drug Administration placed restrictions on the use of silicone implants in the U.S., and the use of saline-filled implants has become more common as a result.

Evaluation of the Breast with Prosthesis

Ultrasound evaluations of breasts with prostheses are carried out for two reasons:
- **The examination of the prosthesis for possible complications.**
- **The study of the gland itself for pathology** (either caused by the implant or arising for other reasons).

Two different techniques are used for positioning prostheses:

1) **Retroglandular placement** (fig. 9.1).
2) **Retropectoral placement** (fig. 9.2).

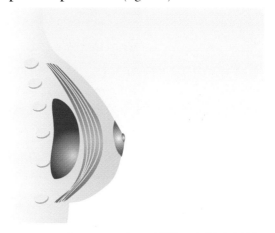

Figure 9.2

Frequently after implant surgery a layer or capsule of fibrous connective tissue forms around the implant. This is generally a thin band of tissue, poorly supplied, and separated spatially from the prosthsis. It may be found in 20% of breast implants (the percentage being less in retropectoral prostheses).

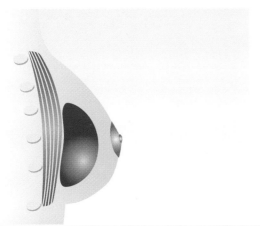

Figure 9.1

Retropectoral implants have two main disadvantages: they present a greater chance of upward migration, causing pain during physical exertion, and some studies suggest they may increase long term chances of glandular ptosis.

In normal conditions the mammary layers described in

Chapter 1 may be evaluated by ultrasound. Evaluation of the prosthesis itself should concentrate on:
- **The borders, which are generally thin, well-defined, highly echogenic.**
- **The contents, which are anechoic** (as is any liquid).

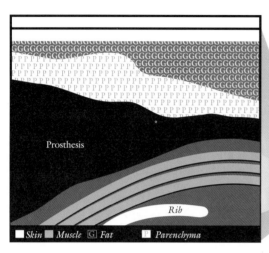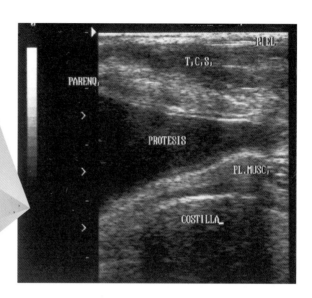

Figure 9.3 Image displaying the following anatomical layers: skin, subcutaneous cell tissue, mammary parenchyma, implant capsule consisting of fibrous tissue (echogenic band), silicone implant (anechoic band), muscle layer, and rib cage.

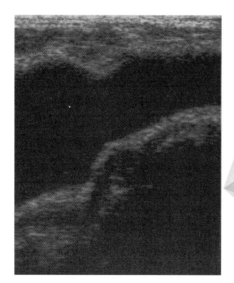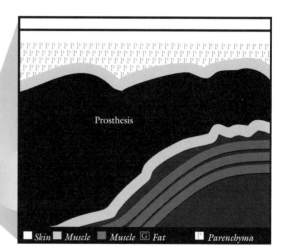

Figure 9.4 Image of the following layers in a patient with a retroglandular implant: skin, subcutaneous cell tissue, a small area of mammary parenchyma, capsule consisting of fibrous tissue showing small, insignificant irregularities, silicone implant (anechoic), muscle layer, rib cage.

In some cases and depending on the patient and the equipment used, an artifact or reverberation (which should not be confused with a pathology) will appear as a fine band of echoes near the border of the implant.

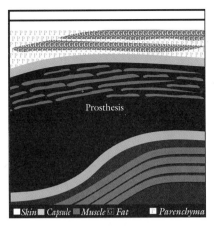

Figure 9.5 Image of a retroglandular-located implant. Beneath the capsule of fibrous connective tissue (the double echogenic line) an artifact (reverberation) composed of fine, medium intensity echoes can be seen.

□ *Skin* ■ *Capsule* ■ *Muscle* Ⓖ *Fat* Ⓟ *Parenchyma*

Prosthesis

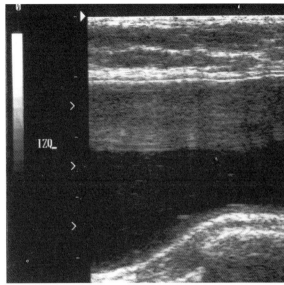

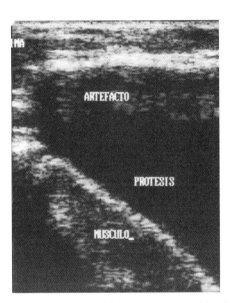

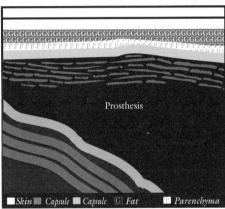

Prosthesis

□ *Skin* ■ *Capsule* ■ *Capsule* Ⓖ *Fat* Ⓟ *Parenchyma*

Figure 9.6 Image of an artifact in the anterior portion of an implant. The reverberation appears as a band of small, heterogeneous echoes along the superficial edge of the implant.

At times folds are produced in the implant which appear in ultrasound images as echogenic lines within the anechoic implant. These folds should not be considered complications.

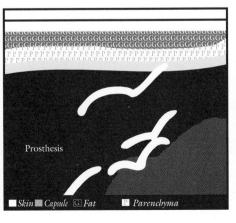

Prosthesis

□ *Skin* ■ *Capsule* Ⓖ *Fat* Ⓟ *Parenchyma*

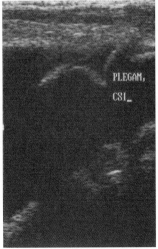

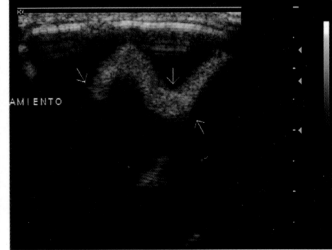

Figure 9.7 Image of a retroglandular-located implant whose contents are anechoic and display a lineal echogenic image in the shape of a seagull.

The diffusion of small quantities of silicone is common, but no conclusive scientific evidence has been produced to confirm that this is dangerous. At times the diffusion of silicone appears sonographically as "snow storms" caused by numerous small echoes of medium intensity.

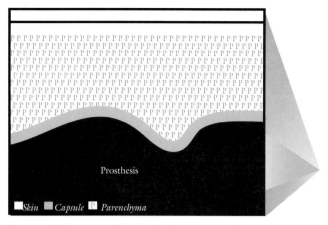
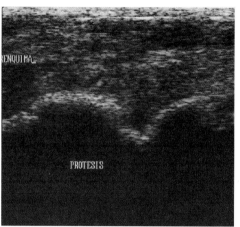

Figure 9.8 Image of an anechoic implant with an irregular hyperechogenic capsule on its surface, and a centrally-located hypoechoic area which is an external diffusion of silicone.

Complications from the Use of Implants

- **Hematomas or abscesses**, which are due to the surgical procedure and appear early in the post-surgical period (see Chapter 8).
- **Displacement of the prosthesis.**

Displacement of the prosthesis occurring shortly after surgery is generally due to the implantation pocket being too small. Displacements that take place much later (which is frequently the case in displacements of retropectoral implants) are caused by the contraction of the capsule of fibrous connective tissue surrounding the implant, which can cause the prosthesis to move upward.

In some cases a short time after the implant surgery the tissues at the level of the incision thin considerably, sometimes to such a degree as to allow one to see the surface of the implant. This requires a second surgical procedure in order to either replace or explant the prosthesis. This is a rare complication, most often observed in patients who have previously undergone mastectomies.

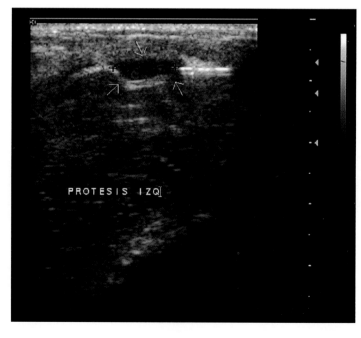

Figure 9.9 Image of an implant displaying fine interior echoes and an irregularity on the surface surrounded by a collection of liquid caused by diffused silicone.

Complications in the Implant Itself

The following complications may be encountered during ultrasound examinations:

1) Retraction of the capsule due to scarring.

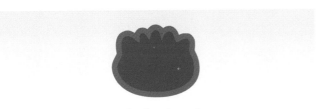

Indented borders and a hard consistency

Figure 9.10

2) Herniation of the implant.

Lobulation of the edge of the implant without rupture

Figure 9.11

3) Extracapsular rupture.

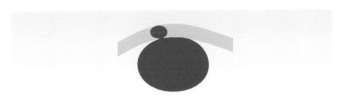

Silicone leaks into adjacent tissues

Figure 9.12

4) Extracapsular rupture with fine echoes.

Silicone leaks into adjacent tissue and the implant contains fine echos.

Figure 9.13

5) Intracapsular rupture.

The silicone is contained within the fibrotic capsule and echogenic lines may appear within the implant

Figure 9.14

6) Intracapsular and extracapsular rupture.

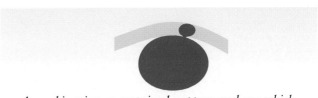

A combination: a contained rupture and one which leaks into the adjacent tissues.

Figure 9.15

The rupture of a prosthesis and subsequent leakage of silicone is an infrequent complication (5-8%), generally caused by trauma. It is still unclear if exposure to silicone is dangerous, but loose silicone in the breast can form granulomas. A rupture should be suspected if any of the following signs are encountered:

- **Mammary asymmetry.**
- **A decrease in implant tension.**
- **A decrease in mammary volume.**
- **Palpable silicone nodules (which must be differentiated from other types of nodules).**

Spontaneous ruptures are most frequent approximately 10 years after the placement of the implant. Notably, hydrogel-filled implants tend to absorb fluids upon rupture, and this may cause breast volume to increase. Ultrasound allows evaluation of both the implant and the overlying parenchyma, and therefore is one of the few methods available for detecting ruptures.

Contraction of the encapsulation of fibrous connective tissue occurs in 10 to 20% of women and can occur weeks or years after placement. Contracted implants become hard, deform, and may cause pain.

Older prostheses may have fibrotic encapsulations which contain a number of calcium deposits of various sizes.

According to Destouet, 17% of implants develop herniations, which are lobulations of the implant without rupture or leakage.

In cases of ruptured implants requiring surgery it is important to determine what type of rupture has occurred and where the contents of the implant are contained. If the leakage is contained within the encapsulation the surgical procedure will be less complicated and the implant can be removed without diffusion of silicone into the parenchyma.

Ultrasound images of ruptured prostheses will show leaking silicone and will possibly display multiple small echoes which are caused by the mixture of silicone and organic elements near the rupture.

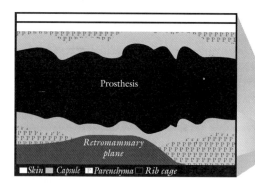

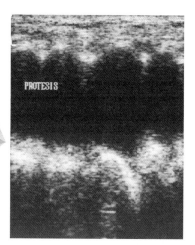

Figure 9.16 Image of a retroglandular implant displaying a strong echogenic reaction and multiple surface irregularities due to retraction of the encapsulation of fibrous connective tissue.

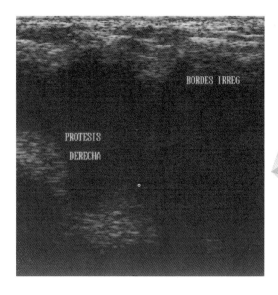

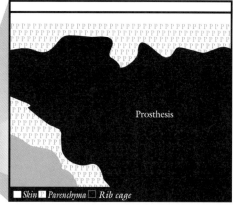

Figure 9.17 Image of an implant with a herniation in a patient complaining of a palpable deformation of the implant.

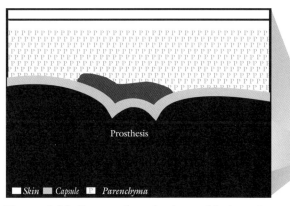

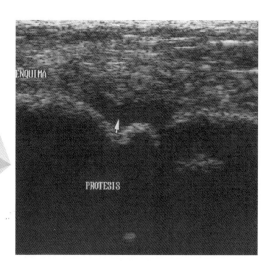

Figure 9.18 Image of an implant with irregular borders displaying an anechoic area of diffused silicone possibly caused by a rupture in the implant.

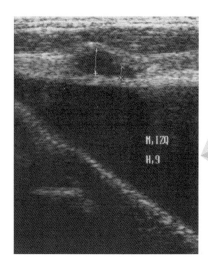

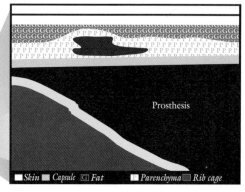

Figure 9.19 Image of an elongated anechoic area in front of the implant caused by a collection of silicone which emerged from a rupture in the implant.

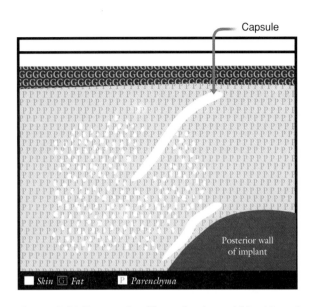

Capsule

Posterior wall
of implant

Skin G Fat P Parenchyma

Figure 9.20 Image of a silicone implant within thinned mammary parenchyma. The implant displays fine interior echoes and an echogenic band along the edge of the capsule which was determined to be a fold.

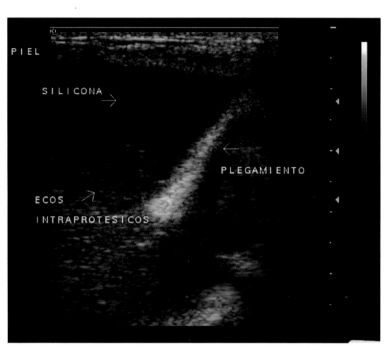

PIEL

SILICONA

PLEGAMIENTO

ECOS
INTRAPROTESICOS

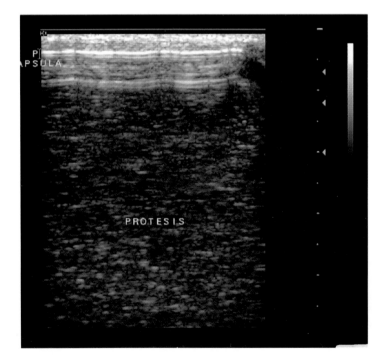

PIEL
CAPSULA

PROTESIS

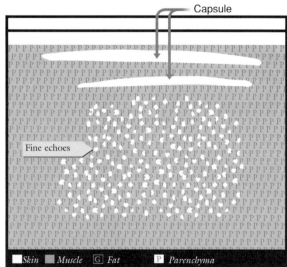

Capsule

Fine echoes

Skin Muscle G Fat P Parenchyma

Figure 9.21 *(Figs. 9.21-9.24 are of the same silicone implant)* Image of an implant displaying a double capsule and fine interior echoes. This area shows no signs of rupture.

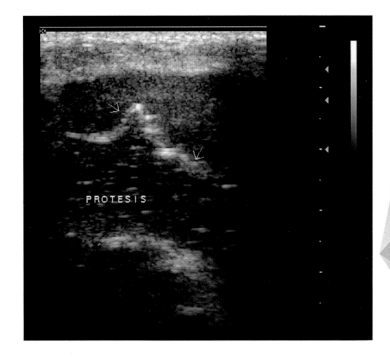

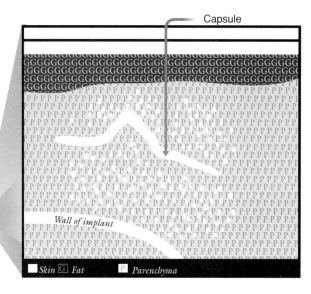

Figure 9.22 Image of the implant showing signs of folding and fine interior echoes.

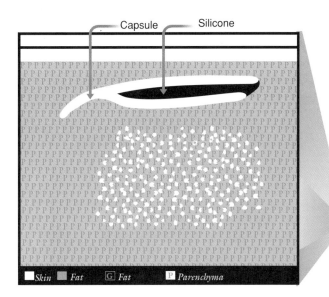

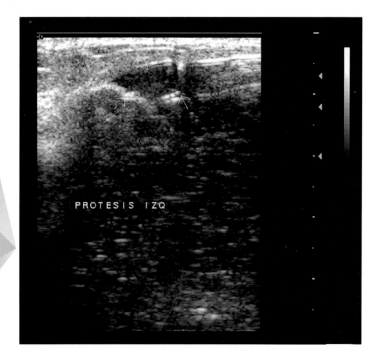

Figs. 9.23, 9.24 Two different views of the same section of the implant which show an irregularity and signs of rupture with silicone on both sides of the implant.

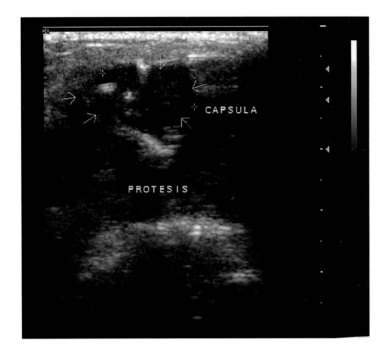

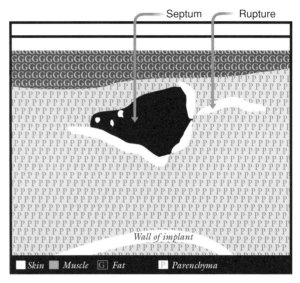

Figure 9.24

Evaluation of the Parenchyma in Patients with Implants

An examination of breasts with prostheses should consider the possibly of both:

- **Pathologies inherent in the gland itself** (either benign or malignant).
- **Pathologies resulting from the presence of uncontained silicone within the parenchyma.**

In cases of pathologies inherent in the gland itself the same procedures for the analysis of breasts without prostheses should be followed. Ideally, the patient will have a record of examinations carried out before the implant surgery which will provide a basis for comparison or correlation. In questionable cases one should not hesitate to perform a US-guided puncture, which allows a timely, decisive diagnosis without danger of damaging the prosthesis.

Ultrasound images are also useful in cases of non-palpable pathologies which require exploratory surgery, because they aid in establishing the exact location of the prosthesis.

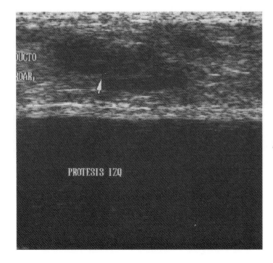

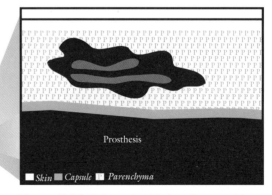

Figure 9.25 Galactophoritis in a breast with an implant.

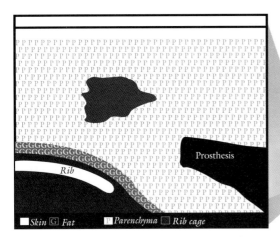

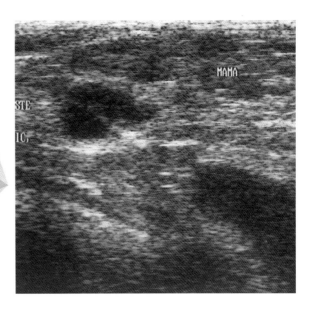

Figure 9.26 Image of a hypoechoic mass displaying defined borders and a septum near the axillary tail of the breast and outside the implant itself. It was diagnosed as a cyst with a septum.

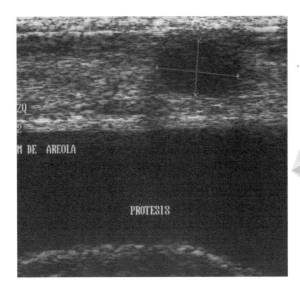

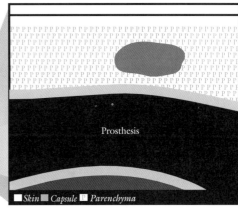

Figure 9.27 Image of a hypoechoic mass with partially defined borders in the middle of the parenchyma of the superior quadrant, 4cm from the areola. Medular carcinoma.

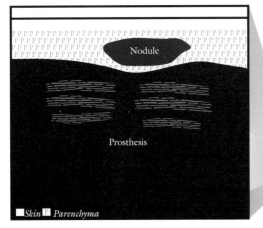

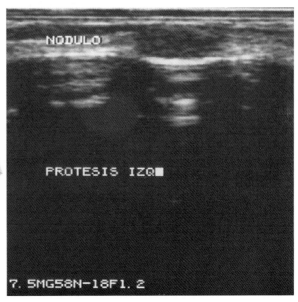

Figure 9.28 Image of a solid, hypoechoic mass within low-volume mammary parenchyma, in contact with the skin and displaying low echogenicity and defined borders. It was diagnosed as a fibroadenoma.

In a study of 35 women with both breast implants and breast cancer, Silverstein et al. found that 97% had palpable lesions. This suggests that women with prostheses should follow the same strict schedule of screenings as women without implants, or undergo more frequent screenings.

Although mammography is the best method for early diagnosis, one must consider that implants reduce the visibility of the parenchyma by 50% (visibility may be increased to 60-65% by using the Eklund manuever, simultaneously pulling the gland forward while keeping the implant in place. Retropectoral implants allow 90% visibility of the parenchyma in most cases). Due to this reduced visibility it is advisable to perform periodical combined check-ups in order to optimize diagnosis.

Injection of Free Silicone

The injection of free silicone into the breast for augmentation purposes also results in poor visibility. In these cases the parenchyma (and any pathologies therein) is severely distorted or blocked from view by the presence of silicone.

The ultrasound image produced is heterogenic, with strong echoes and shadows, and will generally display numerous lacunae on the various tissue layers.

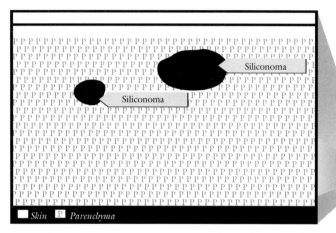

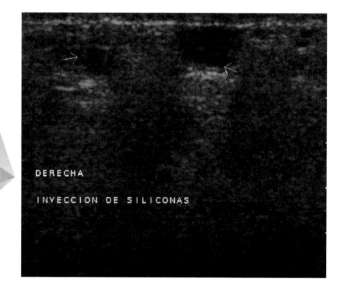

Figure 9.29 Image of siliconomas (pseudocysts) in a patient who had received a free injection of silicone. Both breasts display multiple hypoechoic nodular images, and the anatomic layers are obscured by "snow" caused by fine polymorphic echoes.

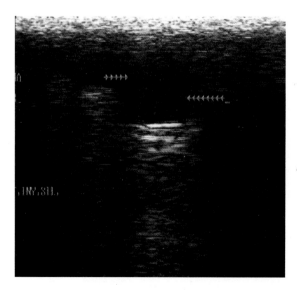

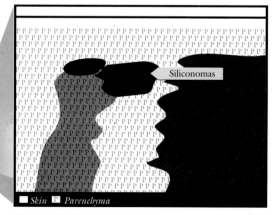

Figure 9.30 Image of "snow" and anechoic masses, some with sonic enhancement on the posterior wall due to the injection of silicone.

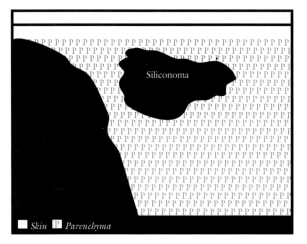

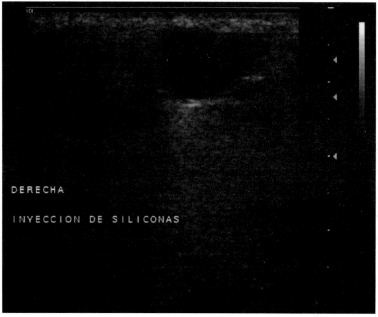

Figure 9.31 Image of an anechoic mass in contact with the skin which is a siliconoma formed from encapsulated silicone. The mammary layers are obscured as an effect of the free injection of silicone.

References

- Cramer, L. M. y colaboradores. The Living Link, A Necessity for Successful Implantation. Transact. Fifth International Congress. Plastic Surgery. Butterworths, Australia, 1971, pp. 776.
- Cronin, T. DD. et al. Augmentation Mammaplasty: A New "Natural Feel" Prosthesis. Transact. Third International Congress. Plastic Surgery. Excepta Medica Foundation. Amsterdam, 1964, pp. 41.
- De Camara, L. D. y colaboradores. Rupture and Aging of Silicone Gel Breast Implants. PRS, 1993; 9 (5); 828-834.
- Miller III, A. et al. A Nine Year Prospective Study of Immunologic Related Diseases in Implated Patients. Abstract from the American Society of Plastic and Reconstructive Surgery's 63rd Annual Scientific Meeting. San Diego, 1994.
- Peters, W. J. Factors Affecting the Rupture of Silicone Gel Breast Implants. Annals of Plastic Surgery, 1994; 33(4): 462-463.
- Slaving, S.A. et al. Silicone Gel Implant Explanation: Reasons, Results, and Admonitions. PRS, 1995; 95 (1): 63-69.

10

Sequelae and Recurrence in the Breast Treated for Cancer

M. E. Lanfranchi

Introduction

Before 1980, when the normal treatment for breast cancer was mastectomy, follow-up was generally limited to the skin, the ribcage, and the contralateral breast.

This changed however, with the advent of conservative surgical techniques. These techniques increase the quality of life for the patient, but also require a more involved follow-up, using both ultrasound and mammography.

Breast cancer may manifest itself as a nodule (see Chapter 5), as microcalcifications, as a disruption in the tissue structure, or as a combination of these; ultrasound (in most cases) can only detect nodules. For this reason mammography combined with an ultrasound examination should be the primary method for diagnosis and follow-up. Since tumors tend to recur in the same form in which they first appeared, this combination of techniques allows for the most complete diagnosis.

If there is in fact a nodule present, it may or may not be palpable. Therefore, it is of utmost importance to arrive at a timely diagnosis, so as to give the patient as many therapeutic options as possible.

Examination Outline

The following is an outline of a follow-up examination:

1) Anamnesis
- Age.
- Post-surgical interval.
- Post-radiotherapy interval.
- Existence of post-surgical complications.
- Anatomical-pathological report.
- If surgery was due to a nodule or microcalcifiactions.

2) Physical Examination
- Point out scars or retractions.
- Mark indurations.
- Check for edema or any other signs.

3) Mammographical Analysis
- Examine previous studies.
- See if there is a correlation between the physical findings and the mammography.
- Make record of the presence of nodules or microcalcifications.

4) Ultrasound Examination
- Examine previous studies.
- Point out scars or other clinical findings.

It is important not only to rule out the possibility of recurrence, but also to be familiar with the modifications which can occur in breasts treated for cancer, in order to avoid diagnostic errors.

Benign Lesions

Benign lesions may occur at any point in the breast, from the surface to the underlying muscle layer. Most lesions involve more than one layer.

a) Affecting the Skin

- **Thickening.**
- **Thinning.**
- **Retraction.**

Thickening of the skin is often seen in the first months of the post-surgical period. It is especially common in radiotherapy and may last six to eight months or longer.

Thinning is generally a sequela which occurs late in the post-surgical period. Retraction is frequently associated with fibrosis of the underlying layers (and displays significant sonic attenuation).

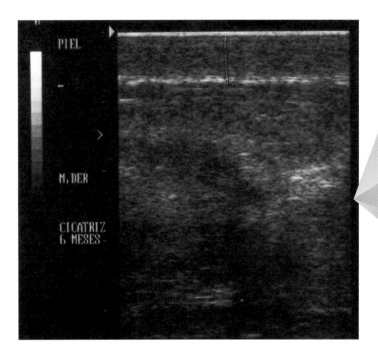

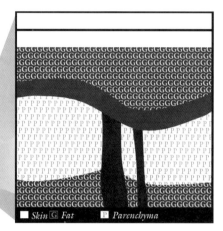

Figure 10.1 Breast of a patient who had undergone surgery to remove a tumor six months before. Image shows an increase in skin thickness due to edema and destruction of the parenchyma as a result of the surgery.

b) Superficial Fascia

May appear normal or may display structural damage as a result of the surgical procedure:

Echogenicity:
- **Decreased:** Caused by fibrosis or edema.
- **Increased:** As a result of radiotherapy.

c) Parenchyma

Damage to the parenchyma may manifest itself as:

- **Disruption** of one or more layers.
- **Modification** of the echogenicity.
- **A pseudonodular** image.

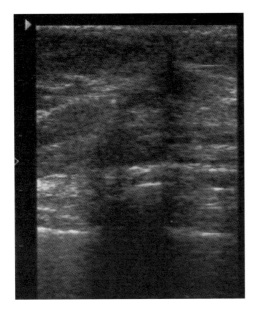

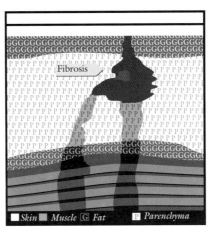

Figure 10.2 Breast of a patient who had undergone conservative surgery 5 years before. Image shows a hypoechoic area originating at the skin level compatible with fibrosis and a posterior nodular image with an echogenic center. It was diagnosed by core biopsy as a post-surgical granuloma.

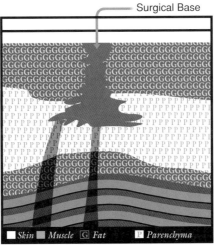

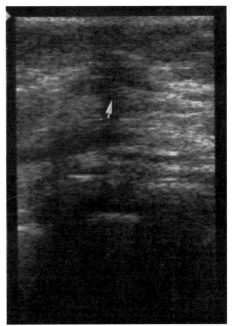

Fig. 10.3 Image of post-surgical fibrosis in a patient who had undergone surgery three years earlier. There is a hypoechoic area which begins at the skin and extends through the gland.

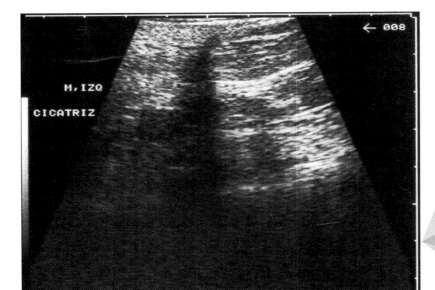

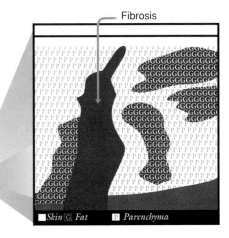

Fig. 10.4 Image of post-surgical fibrosis in a patient with antecedent surgery for infiltrating intraductal carcinoma two years before. Sonic attenuation is observed around the scar due to fibrosis.

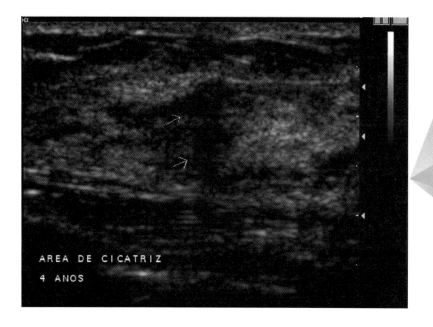

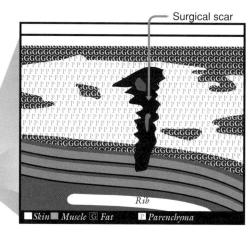

Fig. 10.5 Image of fibrosis in a patient who had undergone surgery four years before. Fibrosis appears along the length of the scar and within the parenchyma.

d) Sequelae due to Radiotherapy

Generally appear as:

- **A decrease in the density of the tissues.**
- **Edema and thickening of the skin.**
- **Distortion in the structure of the tissues.**
- **Increase in the echogenicity of the adipose tissue.**

Microcalcifications are frequently found at the site of the tumorectomy. They are generally visible only by mammography, and require a differential diagnosis between a post-surgical sequela and a recurrence. In the case of a post-surgical sequela the calcifications will be large, thick, and found along the plane of the surgical incision (skin, superficial fascia, and the surgical base). Microcalcifications can appear in 30% of operated breasts, from six months to four years after the completion of radiotherapy. Those which appear early are most often benign.

Other benign calcifications appear in necrotic tissue due to cellular detritus, occur due to fat necrosis, or are produced by the surgical structures.

Calcifications can only be evaluated by ultrasound if they are large; they are normally discovered by mammography and occur in areas of fatty infiltration or in hypoechoic tissue.

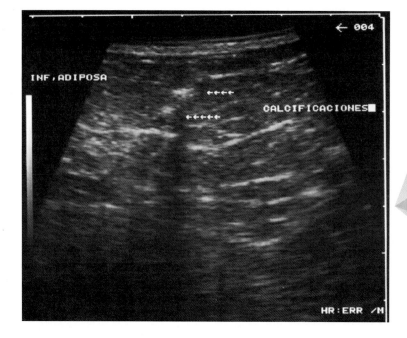

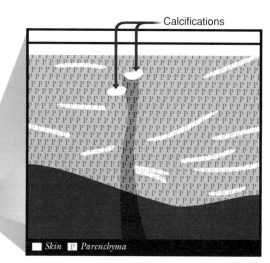

Fig. 10.6 Image of a gland with considerable fatty infiltration and two small calcifications which produce sonic attenuation.

e) Benign Nodular Images

These may be classified according to their echostructure as:
- **Liquid.**
- **Solid.**
- **Complex.**

Anechoic nodular images with a liquid appearance may be caused by:

1) Hematomas:
Unorganized hematomas are homogeneous and lack interior echoes, whereas organized hematomas appear heterogenous.

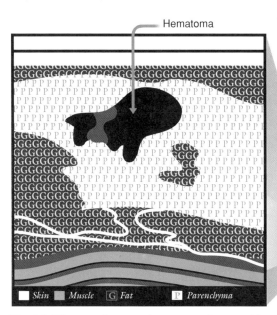

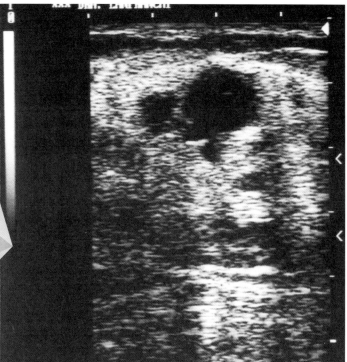

Fig. 10.7 Image of a recent hematoma diagnosed by puncture; it appears as a lobulated anechoic image with a septum.

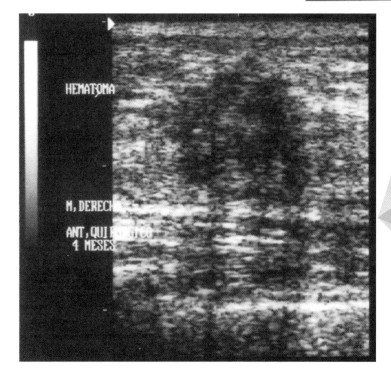

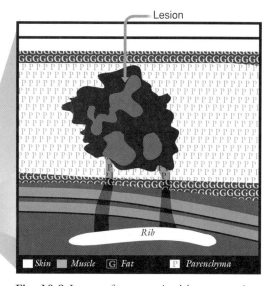

Fig. 10.8 Image of an organized hematoma in a patient who had undergone surgery 4 months before; it appears near the scar as a nodular, heterogeneous image with anechoic areas.

2) Lymphocele or Seroma:

This is a collection of liquid, which may or may not display septations, and which can appear soon after surgery, or up to two years later.

Scar

Lymphocele

☐ Skin ☐ Muscle Ⓖ Fat ☐ Parenchyma

NFOCELE

2 MESES

M, IZQ

H.8

DEBAJO DE CICATRIZ

C.C. 2 MESES

Lymphocele

☐ Skin Ⓖ Fat ☐ Parenchyma

Figs. 10.9, 10.10 Images of lymphoceles in a patient with antecedent conservative surgery for infiltrating ductal carcinoma two months before which appear as liquid anechoic images in the area of the surgical scar.

3) Scar cyst or Oily cyst:

The image is similar to that of a lymphocele, but may display fine interior echoes depending upon its contents.

Cyst

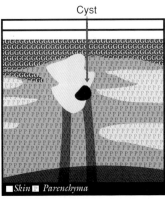

Fig. 10.11 Image of an oily cyst in a patient with antecedent surgery 4 months before; it appears as a small anechoic image.

☐ Skin Ⓟ Parenchyma

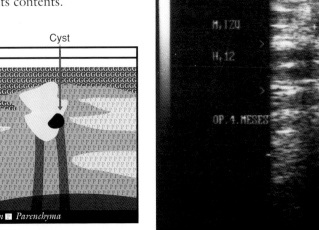

M, IZQ

H, 12

OP. 4 MESES

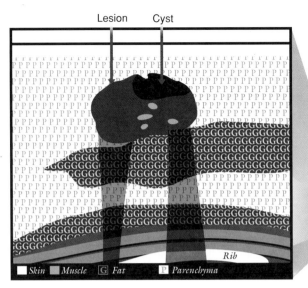

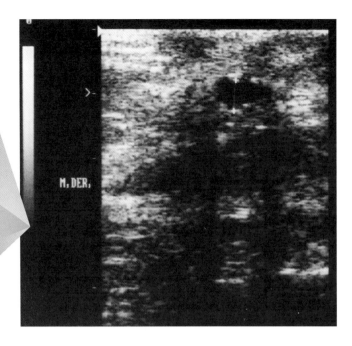

Fig. 10.12 Image of an oily cyst which shows destruction of the tissues and a central anechoic area.

4) Abscess:

The image produced has a liquid appearance and irregular or scalloped borders; abscesses sometimes display fine interior echoes and move if compressed by the transducer (see Chapter 8).

Nodular images with a solid appearance can be divided into three types:

1) Granuloma.
2) Fat necrosis.
3) Calcifications.

Images of granulomas appear solid and can have either homogeneous or heterogeneous echostructure and either regular or irregular borders. Granulomas are typically solid, hypoechoic, and with a central area of increased echogenicity.

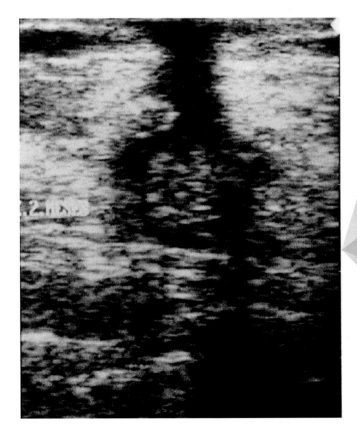

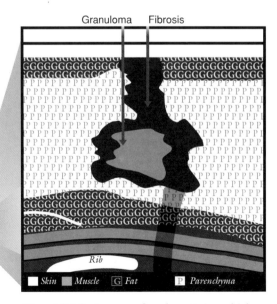

Fig. 10.13 Image of a breast in which a hypoechoic area of fibrosis extends from the skin into the parenchyma. Beyond the fibrosis there is a nodular image with an echogenic center which was diagnosed as a scar granuloma.

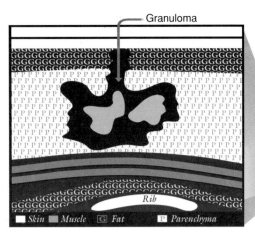

Granuloma

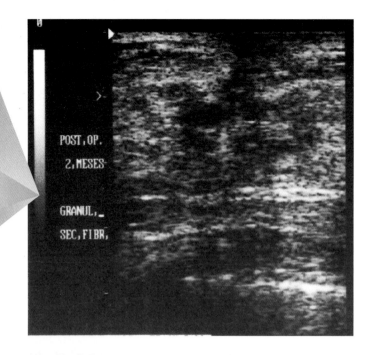

| Skin | Muscle | G Fat | P Parenchyma |

POST, OP.
2, MESES
GRANUL,_
SEC, FIBR,

Fig. 10.14 Image of fibrosis and a benign post surgical granuloma in a patient complaining of a palpable nodule who had undergone surgery 2 months before. Fibrosis appears as a hypoechoic image originating near the skin; granuloma appears as a pseudonodular image with an echogenic center.

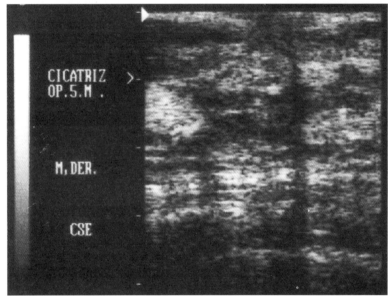

CICATRIZ >
OP.5.M.

M, DER.

CSE

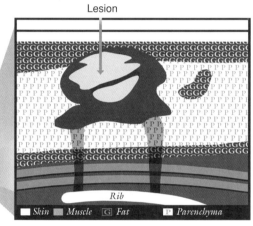

Lesion

| Skin | Muscle | G Fat | P Parenchyma |

Fig. 10.15 Image of fibrosis and a benign post-surgical granuloma in a patient complaining of a palpable nodule who had undergone surgery 5 months before.

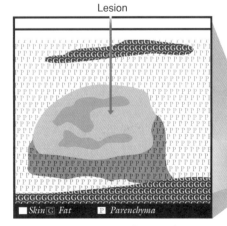

Lesion

| Skin | G Fat | P Parenchyma |

Fig. 10.16 Image of an echogenic benign sequela in a patient complaining of a palpable nodule who had undergone conservative surgery one year before.

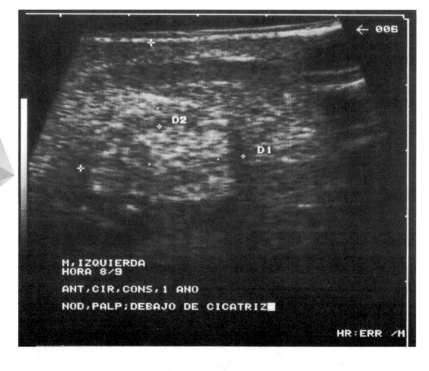

← 006

D2

D1

M, IZQUIERDA
HORA 8/9
ANT, CIR, CONS, 1 ANO
NOD, PALP; DEBAJO DE CICATRIZ■

HR:ERR /M

When one encounters a granuloma with irregular borders or sonic attenuation, it is advisable to perform a differential diagnosis with a tumoral recurrence. A ultrasound-guided (US-guided) cytological or histological puncture is the best method of confirming diagnosis in these cases.

Fat necrosis may appear in the following forms:
- **A solid, heterogeneous image.**
- **A mixed image with both solid and liquid components.**

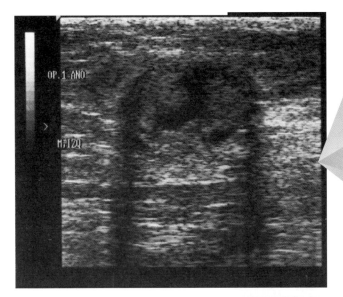

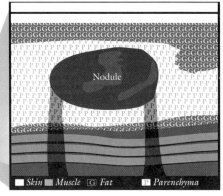

Fig. 10.17 Image of fat necrosis in a patient who had undergone conservative surgery one year before; it appears as a heterogeneous nodule with an echogenic center.

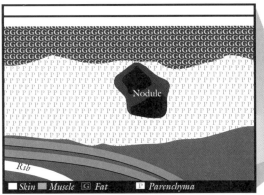

Fig. 10.18 Image of fat necrosis which appears as a hypoechoic nodule with 2 anechoic areas.

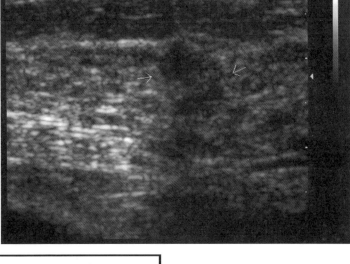

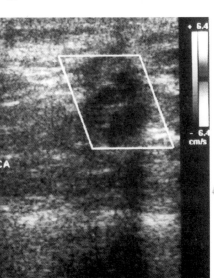

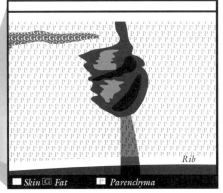

Fig. 10.19 Image of fibrosis and fat necrosis in a patient who had undergone conservative surgery 2 years before; there is sonic attenuation near the scar and 2 hypoechoic areas without echoes.

185

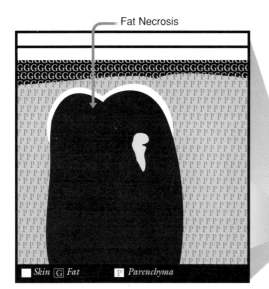

Fat Necrosis

☐ Skin �G Fat ℗ Parenchyma

Fig. 10.20 Image of a breast with 2 areas of considerable sonic attenuation which obscure the structures beneath. It was diagnosed as an area of fat necrosis with calcifications by correlation with a mammographical examination.

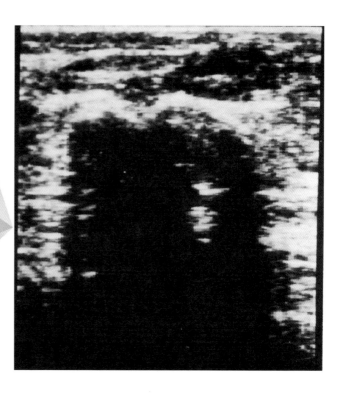

- **A solid image with thick calcifications and significant sonic attenuation** (sonic attenuation of this type is generally encountered only in advanced cases).

In ultrasound images fat necrosis with calcifications and sonic attenuation can be mistaken for a neoplasm. However, it is pathognomonic when observed by mammography; for this reason a combined diagnosis is essential.

The calcifications themselves can be seen by ultrasound if they are voluminous or found within a nodule (within an area of fat necrosis, for example). However, a mammographical examination must be performed in order to examine them and confirm diagnosis.

Ultrasound images of calcifications are always echogenic and display significant sonic attenuation.

Mixed images with both solid and liquid areas are generally abscesses, hematomas, or areas of fat necrosis. Scars will either not appear in ultrasound images or will create carcinoma-like images due to their high degree of fibrosis.

Statistics

Pathologies are arranged by frequency:

Pathology	Frequency
Skin Edema	96%
Skin Retraction	70%
Collections of liquid	35%
Benign Calcifications	30%
Structural Distortion	22%
Fat Necrosis	8%
Granuloma and fibrosis	8%
Scarring	2%

Table 10.1

Frequency of benign pathologies which did not appear in clinical examinations but were found by ultrasound or mammography.

Pathology	Frequency
Benign nodule discovered by ultrasound	54.1%
Benign nodule discovered by mammography	25.47%
Negative mammography and ultrasound	18.89%

Table 10.2

Malignant Lesions

Pathologies encountered during the follow-up period may be:

a) **Residual cancer:** due to insufficient surgical excision (this type is quickly discovered).

b) **Recurrence:** cancers found in or near the surgical base or surrounding areas (one must bear in mind the normal distortion of the parenchyma resulting from surgery).

c) **Cancer of the contralateral breast:** easier to diagnose due to its locus in unaltered parenchyma.

It is important to evaluate the surgical base, as this is the most common location of recurrences. The frequency of recurrences in cases of conservative treatment is between 5 and 10% (6.3% according to our research).

Variations depend upon the stage in which the pathology is discovered and the amount of time which has passed since treatment. Recurrences most frequently occur 36 to 40 months after surgery; 65% are found in the surgical base, 22% near the base, and 13% are multifocal.

According to a study conducted by Stomper et al. 43% of recurrences detected by mammography are in the form of microcalcifications. As previously mentioned, ultrasound can detect nodules, but not these microcalcifications.

Recurrence should be suspected when an ultrasound image of a scar or surgical sequela which has gone unchanged during a number of examinations begins to modify, appearing to form a nodular border.

Recurrences are common in cases in which the original tumor was either a comedocarcinoma or was invasive, with an extensive intraductal component.

The ultrasound image of the recurrence will in most cases be the same as that of the original cancer. Generally these images will be hypoechoic with irregular borders, heterogenic echostructure, and variable sonic attenuation.

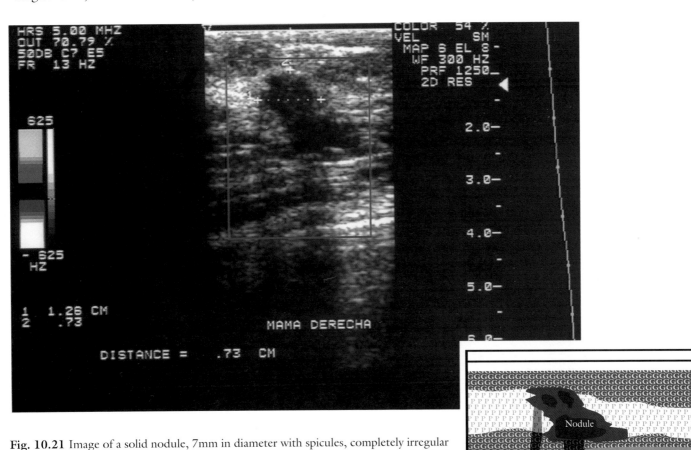

Fig. 10.21 Image of a solid nodule, 7mm in diameter with spicules, completely irregular borders, and its greatest diameter perpendicular to the skin in a patient who had undergone conservative surgery 3 years before. It was diagnosed as a recurrent infiltrating ductal carcinoma.

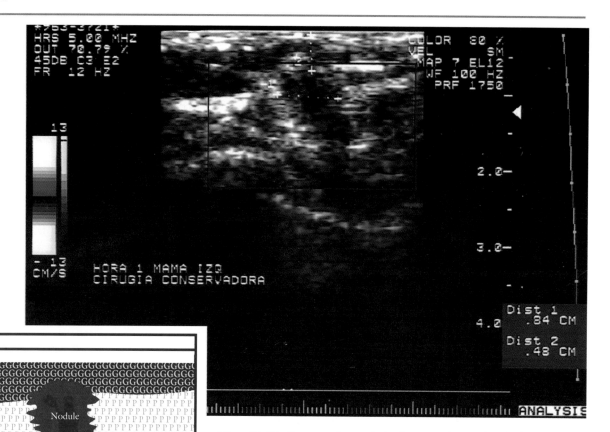

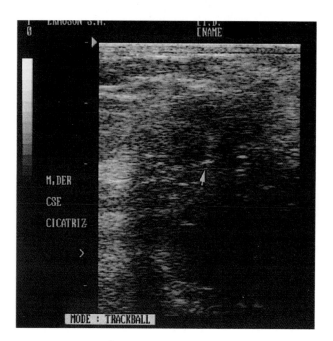

Fig. 10.22 Image of neoplasia in a patient who had undergone conservative surgery 3 years prior; it appears as a solid, heterogeneous nodule with a significant posterior acoustic shadow.

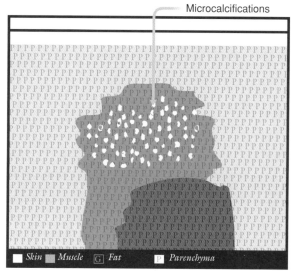

Fig. 10.23 Image of a recurrent comedocarcinoma in a patient who had undergone conservative surgery 18 moths prior; it appears as an area with poorly-defined borders and multiple calcifications.

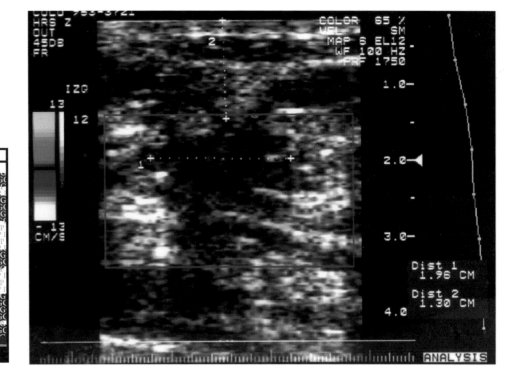

Fig. 10.24 Image of a recurrent tumor in a patient who had undergone conservative surgery 34 months prior; appears as a solid nodule with heterogeneous echostructure and spicules which produces sonic attenuation.

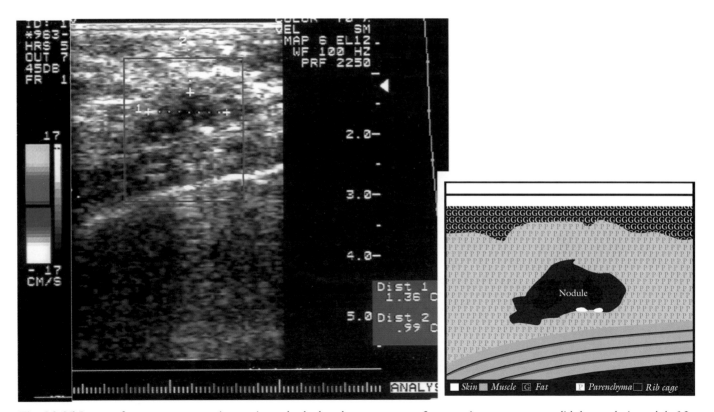

Fig. 10.25 Image of a recurrent tumor in a patient who had undergone surgery 3 years prior; appears as a solid, hypoechoic nodule 13 x 9mm in size with irregular borders and small calcifications.

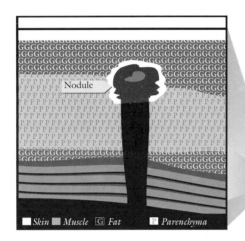

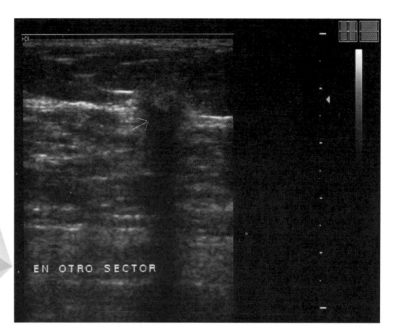

Fig. 10.26 Image of a neoplasia in a patient who had undergone conservative surgery 3 years before; it appears as a solid, heterogeneous nodule with a significant posterior acoustic shadow.

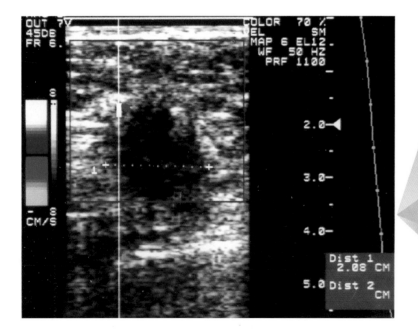

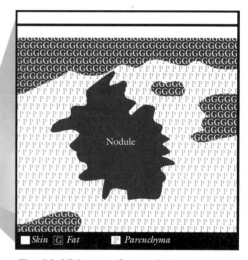

Fig. 10.27 Image of a neoplasia; it appears as a solid, heterogeneous nodule with irregular borders and increased echoes in the surrounding tissues.

In some cases the image of the recurrence may be altered because of its proximity to the surgical scar. The possibility exists that concomitant or simultaneous pathologies, such as combinations of fibrosis and carcinoma, fibrosis and fibroadenoma, or a recurrence combined with fibroadenoma, may also be found during follow-up examinations.

Edema accompanied by thickening of the skin and alterations in the echogenicity of the parenchyma, if encountered soon after treatment, can be attributed to the effects of surgery and radiotherapy. Edema may last for a number of months or up to a year after treatment and then disappear spontaneously.

Using ultrasound one can measure edema in the skin (2-3 mm is normal) as well as monitor the thickness of the skin itself.

If skin thickness diminishes after the edema has disappeared, then stabilizes only to later thicken again gradually, one should rule out the possibility of carcinomatous lymphangitis.

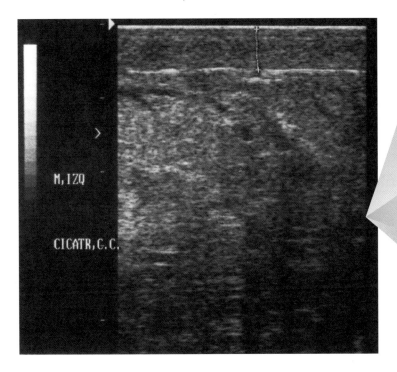

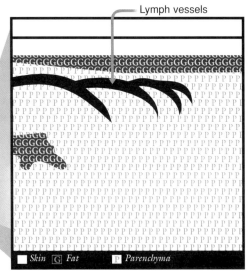

Fig. 10.28 Image of carcinomatous lymphangitis in a patient who had undergone previous conservative surgery; the skin has thickened and there are numerous lineal anechoic images which are the lymph vessels.

Tables 10.3 and 10.4 below show the percentage of recurrences (by type) found by mammography and by ultrasound.

Mammography	
Nodules	30%
Microcalcifications	29%
Glandular Distortion	9%
Increase in density	8%
Negative	24%

Table 10.3

Ultrasound	
Nodules	55%

Table 10.4

In a German study Gerlach presented the following percentages concerning the diagnosis of recurrences:
- **Diagnosed by ultrasound only: 26%**
- **Diagnosed by mammography only: 10%**
- **False positives produced by ultrasound: 17.2%**
- **False positives produced by mammography: 45.5%**

It is worth noting here that currently mammography is the only method capable of detecting microcalcifications.

A study by Stomper states that 35% of relapses were diagnosed by mammography only, and 61% were diagnosed by a combination of physical examination and mammography.

In a French study Balu-Maestro presented the following percentages concerning diagnosis of recurrences:
- **Diagnosed by mammography only: 95.5%**
- **Diagnosed by ultrasound only: 90.9%**
- **Diagnosed by physical examination: 45.5%**

In the author's clinical experience ultrasound is more sensitive than mammography to benign abnormalities (see table 10.5 below).

Benign Abnormalities	
Ultrasound sensibility	95.7%
Mammography sensibility	72.3%
Table 10.5	

For example, in some cases mammography will only detect an opaqueness, whereas ultrasound can confirm or rule out the presence of a nodule.

The breast is a dynamic organ which undergoes modifications after surgery and/or radiotherapy. Since most significant variations occur 6 to 12 months after treatment, a schedule for follow-up exams should be established.

The risk of recurrence increases 1 to 2% each year after treatment, so a US-guided puncture, with either a fine or thick needle, is recommended if the image is not conclusive.

In the author's opinion mammography, in addition to its capability to detect microcalcifiactions, is more effective than ultrasound in ruling out a recurrence in scar tissue or fat necrosis. However, ultrasound is more useful in the diagnosis and follow-up of benign abnormalities and collections of liquid. Also, ultrasound can confirm or rule out the existence of a benign or malignant nodule, whereas mammography will only show an opaque area.

References

- Russo J, Frederick J, Ownby HE, Fine G, Hussain M, Krickstein HI, Robbins TO, Rosenberg B: Predictors of recurrence and survival of patients with breast cancer. *Am J Clin Pathol* 1987; 88:123-131.
- Graverson HP, Blichert-Tolf M, Anderson J A, Zedeler K: Breast cancer: Risk of axillary recurrence in node-negative patients following partial dissection of the axilla. *Eur J Sur Oncol*, 1988; 14:407-412.
- Eberlein TJ, Connolly JL, Schnitt SJ, Recht A, Osteen RT, Harris JT: Predictors of local recurrence following conservative breast surgery and radiation therapy. The influence of tumor size. *Arch Surg*, 1990; 125:771-775.
- Peters ME, Fagerholm MI, Scanlan KA, Voegeli DR, Kelcz F: Mammographic evaluation of the postsurgical and irradiated breast. *Radiographic*, 1988; 8:873-899.
- Leucht WJ, Rabe DR: Sonographic findings following conservative surgery and irradiation for breast carcinoma. *Ultrasound Med Biol*, 1988; 14 (suppl. 1): 27-41.
- Friedman N: The effects of irradiation on breast cancer and the breast. CA, 1988; 38:368-371.
- Rebner M, Pennes DR, Adler DD, *et al.*: Breast microcalcifications after lumpectomy and radiation therapy. *Radiology*, 1989; 172:577-578.
- Mendelson Ellen: *Evaluation of the postoperative breast. The radiologic clinics of North America*, 1992; 107-136.
- Stomper *et al.*: Mammographic detection of recurrent cancer in the irradiated breast. ADR. 1987; 148:39-43.
- SQ. Solin *et al.*: The detection of local recurrance after definitive irradiation for edrly stage carcinoma of the results of breast biopsies performed in previously irradiated breasts. Concer, 1990; 2497-2502.
- Balu-Maestro *et al.*: Ultrasonographic posttreatment follow up of breast cancer patients. *J. Ultrasound Med*, 1991; 10:1.
- Cady B: The breast bland copeland Philadelphia, Saunders. Choice of operation for breast cancer: conservative therapy versus radical procedures, 1991; 753-769.
- Gerlach B, Holzgreve W, Doren M, Schloo R, Louwen F, Tercanli S, Schneider HPG: Efficiency of breast ultrasound for detection of breast cancer recurrences. Eighth International Congress on the Ultrasonic examination of the breast, 1993. Heidelberg, Germany.
- Amy D, Recurrences of breast carcinoma: early echographic diagnosis. Eighth International Congress on the Ultrasonic examination of the breast, 1993. Heidelberg, Germany.
- El Sayed TF, Cox SJ, Ashford RFU: Role of sonomammography in assessment of volume change in primary breast cancer response to adjuvant therapy. Eighth International Congress on the Ultrasonic examination of the breast, 1993. Heidelberg, Germany.

11

Ultrasound-Guided Intervention

M. E. Lanfranchi
R. Rostagno

Introduction

Ultrasound is very successful in locating and triangulating lesions, and can be used to aid the aspiration of cysts, the positioning of needle and wire guides for preoperative location, and large core needle biopsies.

Ultrasound is capable of locating a nodule in three-dimensional space, which aids in determining the best route through which it can be reached.

There are three basic requirements for ultrasound-guided (US-guided) intervention:
-**The proper equipment.**
-**Adequate puncture materials.**
-**A well-trained operator.**

Proper equipment includes a linear transducer of 7.5 MHz or more, as discussed in Chapter 2. There are a number of companies which manufacture wide-band transducers which function between 5 and 10 MHz.

There are also transducers with guides for carrying out punctures which can be set at the necessary angle between the needle and the lesion. However, the authors prefer to insert the needle by hand because it gives one the freedom to choose the best route of approach and allows one to make any maneuvers which may become necessary.

One must consider the fact that the breast will flatten out when the patient is in the supine position. Precision is of the utmost importance, because of the danger of penetrating the pleural space.

If the lesion is superficial, it is best to insert the needle close to the edge of the transducer using an angle which provides the shortest route to the lesion (see figs. 11.2 and 11.3).

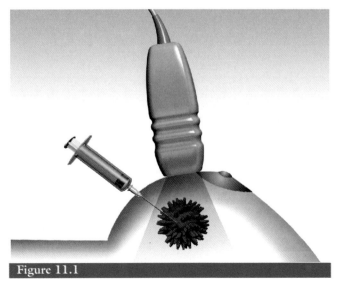

Figure 11.1

Three elements to bear in mind: 1) Location of the nodule. 2) Position of the transducer. 3) Location of the needle.

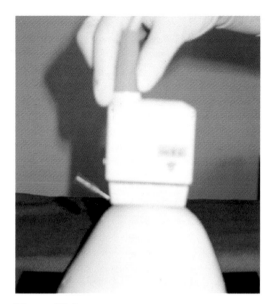

Figure 11.2

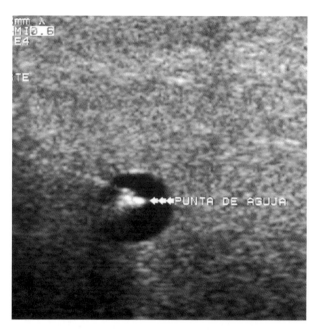

Figure 11.3

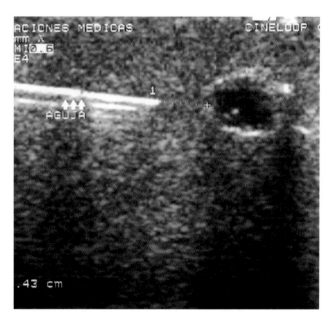

Figure 11.4

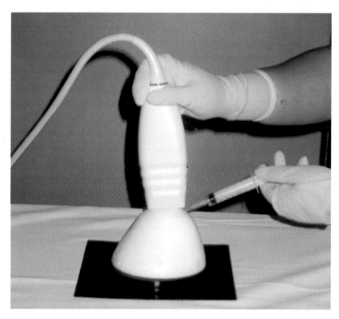

Figure 11.5

If the nodule is located deep within the parenchyma the safest method is to insert the needle at a greater distance from the transducer and as close to parallel to the rib cage as possible (figs. 11.4 and 11.5).

It is advisable to use a phantom until one is completely comfortable with the technique. Phantoms designed for ultrasound are available which have simulated lesions and are similar in form and size to the average breast (figs. 11.5 and 11.8).

The objectives of phantom training are:
- **To become apt at locating lesions and orienting in three-dimensional space.**
- **To become proficient at needle insertion.**
- **To be able to use the transducer to locate and maneuver the needle.**

The needle may be indentified by viewing either its tip or its trajectory. This depends upon which border of the transducer the needle is inserted nearest; needle tips inserted near the long edge generally appear as small, needle-shaped echogenic images (figs. 11.3 and 11.4).

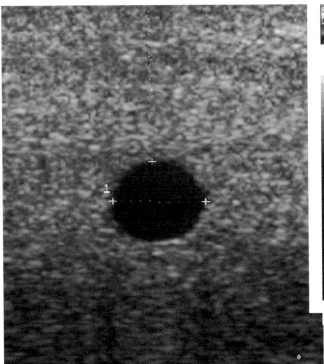

Figure. 11.6 Image of a phantom with a cystic lesion.

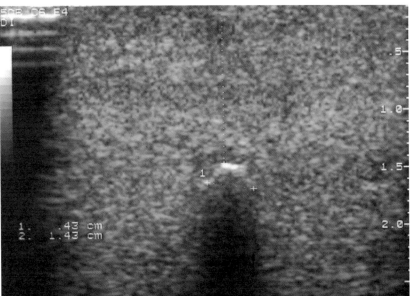

Figure. 11.7 Image of a phantom with a solid, calcified lesion.

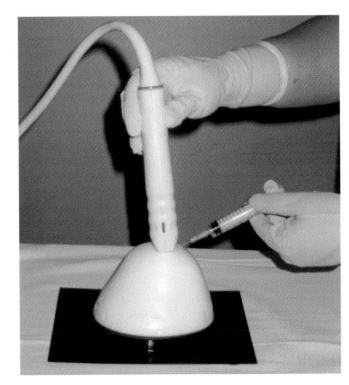

Figure 11.8

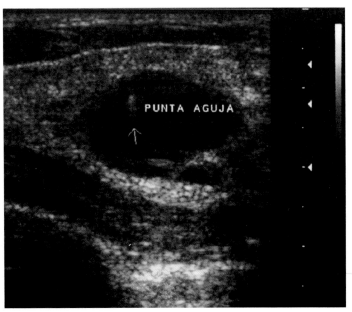

Figure 11.9

However, if the needle is inserted near the short edge it will appear as a lineal echographic image.

Inserting the needle near the short edge is the preferred method, as it allows directional corrections to be made while carrying out the procedure (due to the angle at which the needle and lesion are viewed).

Intervention must be performed by a team of at least two people: one controls the transducer and inserts the needle while the other works the equipment controls and locates the lesion within the breast.

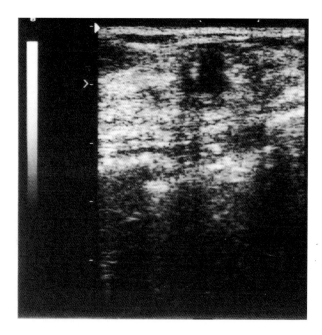

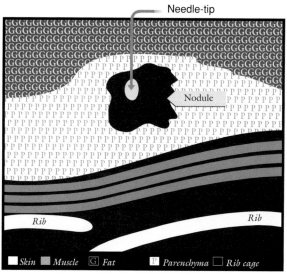

Figure. 11.10 Images of needle puncture of solid and cystic nodules.

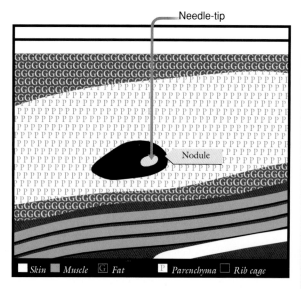

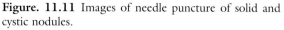

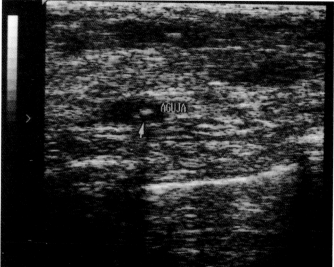

Figure. 11.11 Images of needle puncture of solid and cystic nodules.

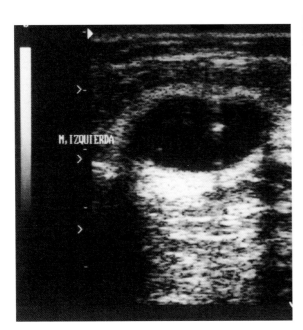

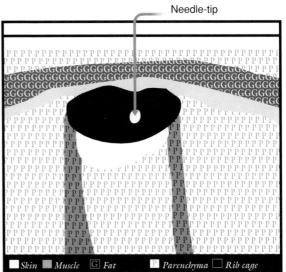

Needle-tip

☐ *Skin* ■ *Muscle* Ⓖ *Fat* ℗ *Parenchyma* ☐ *Rib cage*

Figure. 11.12 Images of needle puncture of solid and cystic nodules.

Types of Ultrasound-Guided Intervention

1) Diagnostic.
2) Therapeutic.
3) Pre-surgical.

1) US-Guided Diagnostic Intervention

This includes any type of intervention for the purpose of collecting a cell or tissue sample in order to determine the etiology of a lesion.

Therefore, diagnostic interventions may be:

a) Cytological.

b) Histological.

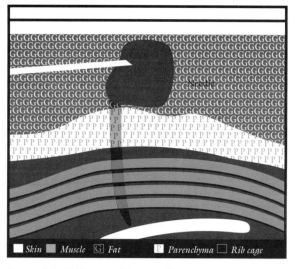

Figure. 11.13 Image of fine needle puncture of a poorly-defined solid nodule.

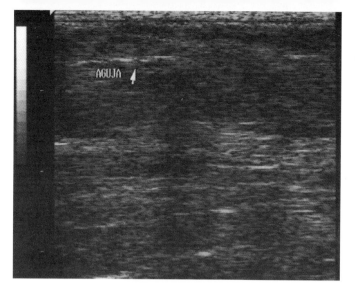

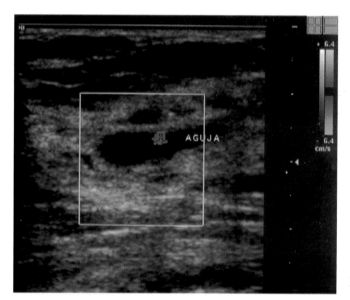

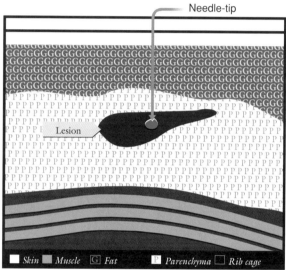

Figure. 11.14 Color Doppler image of needle movement.

One should follow the same basic procedures in preparing for either type of diagnostic intervention:

a) Preparation of the patient:
-Inform her about the technique to be used.
-Explain the reason why it is carried out.

b) Preparation of the breast for puncture:
-Choose the best procedure.
-Carry out an ultrasound study and locate the lesion, in order to select the most convenient route of approach.
-Disinfect the skin (Eg. Yodopovidona).
-Disinfect the transducer (with the corresponding spray).
-Use a sterile gel to carry out the study.

c) Considerations in the selection of materials:
-Depends upon whether the intervention is for:

1) The diagnosis of a solid nodule.
2) The purpose of collection of cells or tissue.
3) Pre-surgical location and/or marking.

It is advisable to place all the necessary materials on an auxilliary table before carrying out the procedure.

For a cytological puncture it is necessary to have the following:
- **10 ml syringes.**
- **A device which provides good negative pressure.**
- **21 G caliber needles.**
- **A clean slide.**

If the cytopathologist is not present at the moment of the puncture and the material must be sent to them it should be fixed with alcohol or an aerosol spray after the smear is made.

Samples should be taken from solid lesions in the following cases:

-Ultrasound images which are inconclusive as to the malignancy of a lesion (hypoechoic masses of very low echogenicity) and have patterns similar to those of complex cysts, fibroadenoma, or medular type circumscript carcinoma.

-A nodule suspected of malignancy, in order to confirm diagnosis and plan therapy.

-Ultrasound images indicating malignancy which contradict mammographical or clinical diagnoses.

-Discovery of multiple masses, either multi-focal (in the same quadrant) or multi-centric (in different quadrants) which could necessitate a change in the therapeutic plan.

-In adolescent or very old patients with images compatible with fibroadenoma, when one must choose to follow the condition or operate.

-Any type of solid nodule that appears during pregnancy.

Technique

- The lesion is located and pinpointed.
- The needle is inserted into the lesion. Its should be moved in and out of the nodule in order to provoke a microtrauma, and a release of the cellular material to be collected. The material can be obtained by aspiration, or by leaving the needle in place for a few moments so that the cells enter the needle due to capillary tension. A smear is then made.

It is advisable to repeat this technique a number of times, making smears of samples taken from various sectors of the nodule, limiting oneself to solid sectors without necrosis.

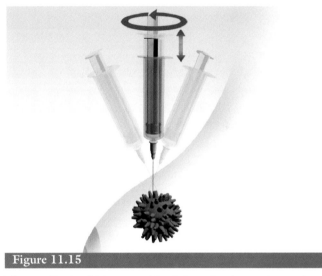

Figure 11.15

The needle should be moved both in a circular motion and up and down within the nodule.

a) US-Guided Fine Needle Aspiration

Recommendations for fine needle aspiration:
- Obtain sufficient material (between 4 and 5 smears).
- Confirm that the material obtained comes from the area of interest.
- Prepare the sample carefully.
- Have an experienced cytopathologist evaluate the samples.

Cautionary procedures:
- Avoid movements perpendicular to the rib cage if possible to avoid puncturing the pleura.
- If the patient has silicone prothesis take extreme care in both moving the prothesis and performing the aspiration.
- Carefully control the trajectory of the needle.
- Select the route of approach nearest the lesion.

Requirements for the success of the procedure
- An experienced cytologist.
- A doctor trained in ultrasound techniques.
- Trained auxiliary personnel to assist the procedure.
- Maintain both the breast and the nodule in a fixed position.
- Aspirate the material if necessary.
- The doctor, cytologist, and assistant should all be present for the duration of the procedure.

Causes for Failure of the Technique:
- Collection of insufficient material.
- Material taken from the wrong area.
- Incorrect puncture or collection techniques.
- Compact-celled tumors.
- Human error due to lack of experience.

Advantages and Disadvantages of Fine Needle Aspiration:

Advantages:
- Does not require anesthesia.
- Does not produce contraindications or complications.
- Gives immediate results, when the cytopathologist is present during the procedure.

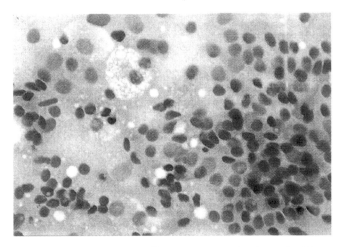

Figure. 11.16 Fine needle puncture aspiration: significant epithelial proliferation, myoepithelial-type bipolar cells, non-suspicious nuclei.

Disadvantages:
- Insufficient or inadequate material in up to the 20% of the cases if the cytopathological results are inconclusive.
- It is necessary to use flawless technique during the procedure and to employ an experienced cytopathologist.

Statistic Results of Fine-Needle Aspiration in Nonpalpable Nodules:

Between January 1996 and December 1998 Rostagno et al. performed 3,837 ultrasound-guided punctures in 2,166 patients with the following statistical results:

Non-Palpable Lesions Cytological Punctures		
Benign Lesions*	2522	92%
Suspicious Lesions	411	15%
Malignant Lesions	137	5%
Insufficient Material	55	2%

Nº 3837
Total # of Pat.: 2166
Jan. 1996-Dec. 1998 . *Cysts: 1730
Table 1

Amongst the benign lesions, 1,730 cases were cysts. The false negatives: (9 cases, or .23%) were:

Non-Palpable Lesions Cytological Punctures False Negatives	
Number of Cases, 2.107 — Jan. 1996 - Dec. 1998	
Infiltrating lobular carcinoma	4
Phyllodes tumor	1
Infiltrating ductal carcinoma	2

Nº 3837
Jan. 1996-Dec. 1998
Table 2

In this population the following was observed:

Non-Palpable Lesions Cytological Punctures	
Sensitivity	95%
Specifity	100%
P.P.V.	100%

Table 3
Following 990 cases for 3 years.

b) US-Guided Histological Puncture (Needle Core Biopsy)

The following materials are required for a histological puncture (needle core biopsy):
- **Puncture equipment; generally pistol-type.**
- **2 or 3 cubic cm of a surface anesthetic.**
- **Small bottles containing formalin in which to place the sample.**

There are various types of pistols for puncture. Some obtain linear sections of tissue, while others produce circular samples.

The needles themselves come in various sizes. The authors prefer to use 14-gauge needles because of the quality of the samples they produce (usually tissue fragments between 15 and 17 mm). One must also be aware that needles come in various lengths, and modify their technique according to the length of the needle used.

Technique

- **The lesion is located and pinpointed.**
- **An assitant holds the breast in place.**
- **The point of the needle should be approximately 9 to 10 mm from the nodule.**

A video recording of the procedure allows one to review the sample collection.

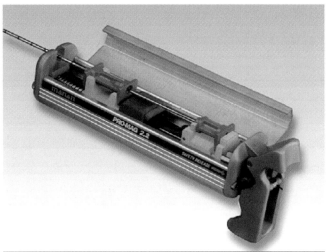

Figure 11.17

Pistol used for needle core biopsies. The main compartment lid is open, displaying the interior. The pistol grip is equipped with both a trigger and a safety.

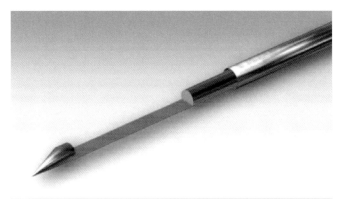

Figure 11.18

Close-up of a needle core biopsy needle showing the recession where the tissue is retained.

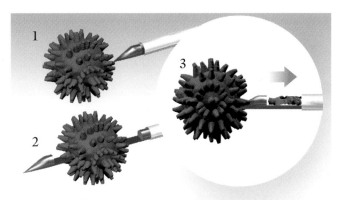

Figure 11.19

Puncture sequence: 1) Pre-shot position. 2) Release of needle within the nodule. 3) Rapid recoil of needle with tissue sample.

Recommendations for Needle Core Biopsies

As in fine needle aspiration, one should repeat the procedure 4 to 5 times in order to obtain sufficient material for the pathologist. If successful this procedure can be used instead of an incisional biopsy in inoperable tumors or when the patient's condition precludes surgery. Figure 11.24 shows an ultrasound image of the collection of a sample.

Advantages and Disadvantages of Needle Core Biopsies

Advantages:
- A larger sample is obtained.
- The histological material is more easily examined by the pathologist.
- It offers the possibility of determining hormone receptors.

Disadvantages:
- It requires local anesthesia and a small incision in the skin at the site of needle penetration.
- Results are not immediate.
- Although rare, it can provoke a hematoma.
- It is not advisable in very small or very deep lesions.
- It is necessary for the radiologist/ultrasound technologist to be trained in the calculation of the pre-shot distance from the tip of the needle to the lesion.
- The patient may display fear or anxiety upon hearing the "shot" (the release of the mechanism).

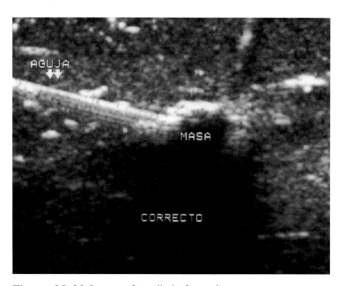

Figure. 11.20 Image of needle before release.

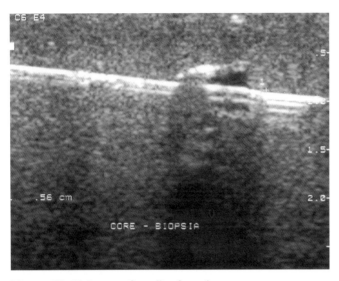

Figure. 11.21 Image of needle after release.

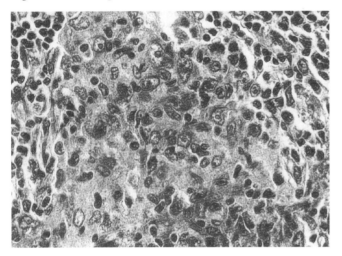

Figure. 11.22 Core needle biopsy sample displaying anastomosis of the large cells with poorly-defined cytoplasmic limits and characteristics indicative of medular carcinoma.

Selection of Puncture Type

One should take into acount:
- **The training of the ultrasound technologist.**
- **Whether a cytopathologist will be present.**
- **The cytopathologist's experience.**
- **The size and location of the lesion.**

Malignant tumors are usually diagnosed as such by cytological and histological punctures. However, cases involving fat necrosis or infiltrating lobular carcinoma are difficult to diagnose by cytological puncture. If these pathologies are present or suspected one should opt for a core needle biopsy.

Table 11.4 shows the number of cytological versus histological punctures performed by the authors.

Cytological Punctures:	**2,741 Patients**	**85%**
Histological Punctures	**485 Patients**	**15%**
Table 11.4		

It is of note that the authors performed numerous core needle biopsies not included in this table because they were cases involving microcalcifications and the biopsies were performed using a stereoatactic guide.

2) Therapeutic Intervention by US-Guided Aspirational Puncture

Therapuetic intervention may be appropriate in the following cases:
- Palpable or non-palpable cystic masses that may cause the patient pain or discomfort.
- Cystic masses with thick or irregular borders.
- Cystic images with apparently thick contents, and fine echoes in suspension (in order to determine contents).
- Collections of liquid or cystic images in patients with silicone implants.
- Puncture and evacuation of post-operatory collections **or** in patients with suspected hematomas.
- Investigation of abscesses (in order to obtain material for a bacteriological study) or galactophoritis.

The same technique used for diagnostic biopsy is used. The caliber of the needle is determined by the characteristics of the liquid as it appears in ultrasound.

If the ultrasound image is of a "clean" liquid without echoes, 21-gauge needles will be sufficient. If the liquid is suspected of being thick, a higher caliber should be used.

Advantage of the Technique
- One has continous control of the procedure until complete evacuation.

Contraindication
- This technique should not be used for cysts with papillary or vegetative contents because once the liquid is evacuated one risks losing the reference point necessary for surgical intervention.

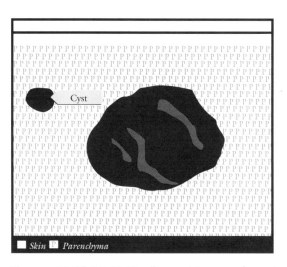

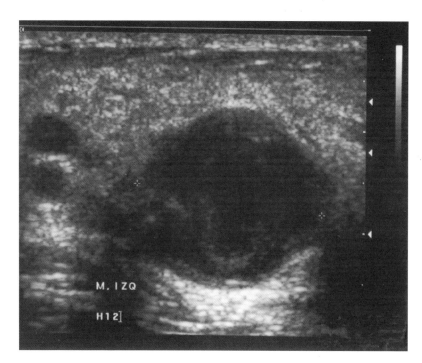

Figures. 11.23-11.28 Needle core biopsy performed on a liquid-filled lesion with irregular echoes.

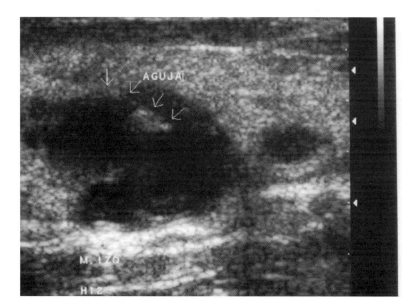

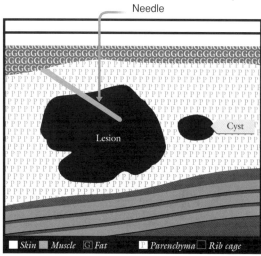

Figure. 11.24 Insertion of the needle.

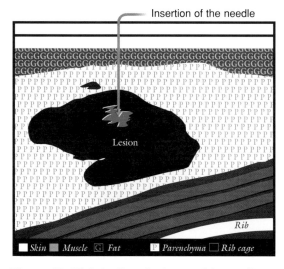

Figure. 11.25 Color Doppler image of the needle tip.

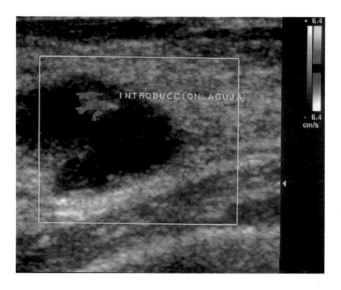

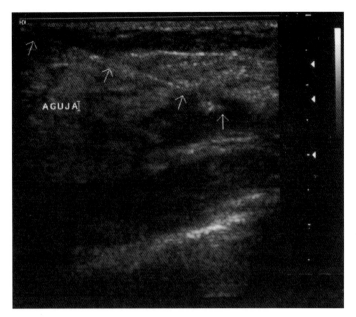

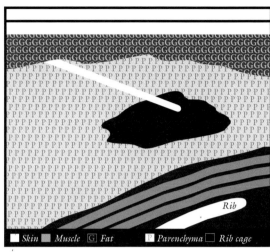

Figure. 11.26 Aspiration until the reduction of the lesion's contents.

3) US-Guided Pre-Surgical Marking

Pre-surgical marking is used in cases of non-palpable lesions. It involves leaving a guide which will aid the surgeon in locating the lesion and facilitates an economical exeresis of tissue.

Pre-Surgical Location and Marking

This technique should be used in the following cases:
- **Any lesion which is non-palpable or not visible by mammography.**
- **A non-palpable lesion located in the axillary tail or deep layers of the breast.**
- **Any non-palpable lesion in a patient with silicone implants.**

The following may be used for marking:
- **Methylene blue.**
- **Medical or inert carbon.**
- **Metallic wire or hooks.**

Methylene blue is easy to use; 1 to 2 mls injected 5 to 10 mm from the lesion are sufficient. It diffuses rapidly however, and should be used within a few hours of surgery. (Carbon may be prefereable in some cases because it does not diffuse as rapidly, allowing it to be placed 48 to 72 hours before surgery).

When methylene blue is injected one should see a corresponding echogenic flash on the screen.

It is advisable to inject the color near, as opposed to within, the lesion in order to avoid causing physical or chemical changes.

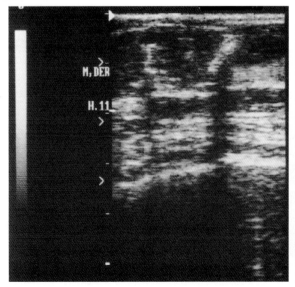

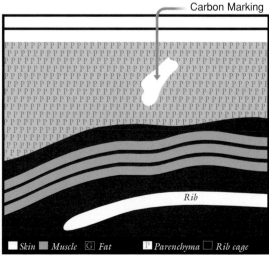

Figure. 11.27 Ultrasound image of carbon marking.

Carbon Marking

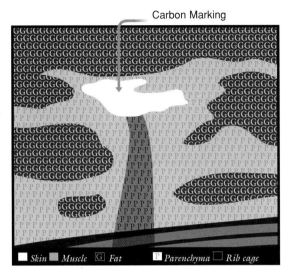

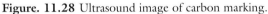

Skin █ Muscle ▣ Fat ᴾ Parenchyma ☐ Rib cage

Figure. 11.28 Ultrasound image of carbon marking.

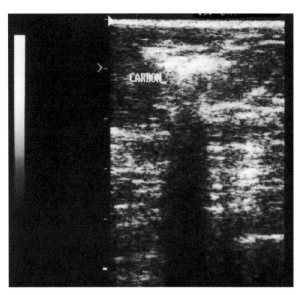

The technique for the insertion of metallic markers is rather simple. The hook and wire are inserted close to the lesion, and then the wire is left projecting from the skin. Care must be taken not to pull or move the wire, in order to avoid breakage. Numerous types of wire of comparable quality are currently available.

A report to the surgeon should be prepared by the doctor performing the marking procedure. It should include:

- **A diagram** showing the exact location of the mark and where it is located in respect to the lesion.

- **A mark** on the skin above the exact location of the lesion, and an exact measurement of the the depth at which it is found.

Advantages and Disadvantages of US-Guided Pre-Surgical Marking

Advantage:
- The lesion can be pinpointed and the marker can be inserted in the exact location desired

Disadvantage:
- Microcalcifications cannot be marked because they are not visible by ultrasound (unless accompanied by a nodule).

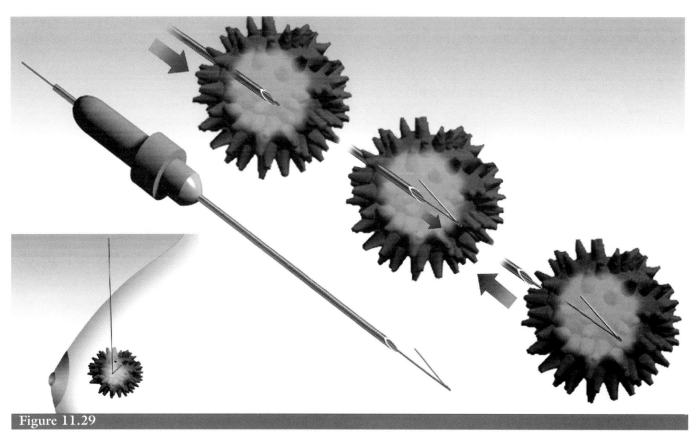

Figure 11.29

These computer images show the insertion of a pre-surgical marking wire and the hook used to mark the non-palpable nodule. Image at bottom left shows the wire protruding from the skin.

Advantages of Guide by Ultrasound Over Guide by Mammography

- The position of the patient is similar to the surgical position.

- Ultrasound is more comfortable because no compression maneuvers need be made.

- It is rapid and reliable in the diagnosis of pathologies located near the rib cage, in the outer quadrants of the breast, and in patients with silicone implants.

- It allows one to choose the most direct route from the skin to the lesion.

- Procedures are conducted in real time, allowing for corrections of the trajectory during the procedure itself.

- Material for cytological or histological study can be extracted from various angles and areas of the lesion.

- Pre-surgical marking can be carried out in the operating room.

Disadvantages of Ultrasound

- Not appropiate for nodules located in breasts with significant fatty infiltration.

- Not appropiate for microcalcifications if they are not combined with a nodule.

Mammotome© System

The Mammotome system guided by stereoatactic mammography has been used since 1994 with very good results, especially in the diagnosis of microcalcifications. Since 1995 the system has also been used with ultrasound, mainly for small nodules.

The system produces samples of at least one gram of tissue, and in many cases only one penetration is needed.

For this reason the Mammotome procedure is more complete and reliable, while being less traumatic, than other methods.

The Mammotome system uses a specially designed needle which cuts, collects, and deposits the sample in a receptacle with the aid of a vacuum (see figs. 11.30 and 11.31).

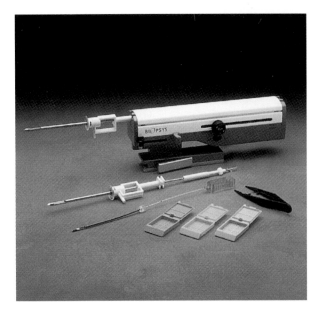

Figure. 11.30

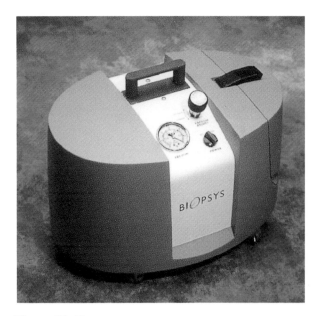

Figure. 11.31

The tissue samples obtained using the Mammotome system are eight times larger than samples obtained with a core biopsy pistol using the same caliber needle (in this case 14-guage; see fig. 11.32).

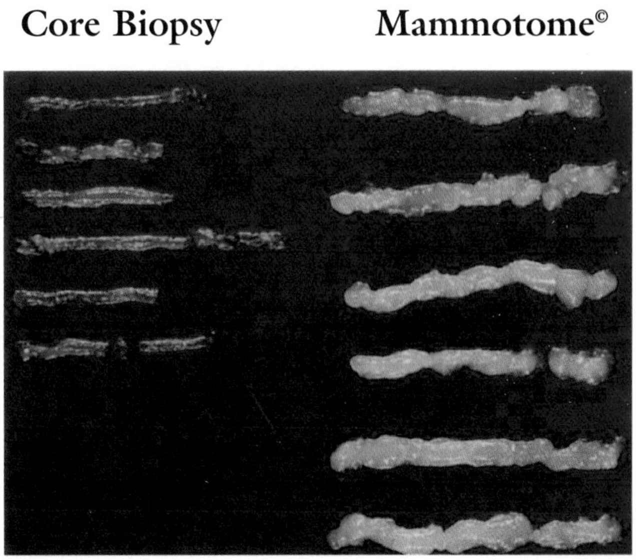

Core Biopsy   **Mammotome©**

Figure. 11.32 Tissue samples with normal core biopsy and with Mammotome.

When the Mammotome needle is inserted into a lesion a rotating cutting cannula pulls the tissue sample into the probe, and then into the collection chamber.

This feature allows one to take samples from different parts of the lesion (or samples of both the mass and the surrounding tissue) without removing the needle (fig. 11.33).

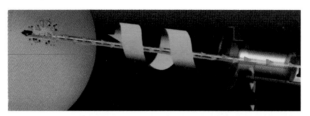

Figure. 11.33 Diagram showing the cutting cannula inserted within a lesion and drawing a tissue sample.

11-gauge needles are recommended for use with the Mammotome system.

If by using this system one extracts all ultrasound evidence of the lesion (i.e. the entire nodule) it is possible to mark the site with metallic clips which can be inserted by the Mammotome catheter itself.

Marking allows for future follow-ups, and/or for surgical excision if the material collected from the nodule is found to be malignant.

A table and a telescoping arm have been developed for the Mammotome which greatly increase the precision with which procedures can be carried out (fig. 11.34).

Using this equipment one holds the ultrasound transducer in one hand while guiding the probe with the other. Once one is prepared to perform the biopsy procedure the arm can be locked into the desired position. In 1997 Burbank et al. published a study concerning non-palpable atypical hyperplasias in which the Mammotome system showed considerable advantages when compared with traditional core needle biopsy procedures.

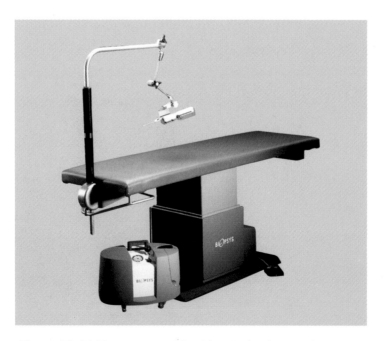

Figure. 11.34 Mammotome table with articulated arm and vacuum chamber.

However, this study was conducted with a Mammotome system guided by mammography. The authors hope that a similar study will soon be conducted using ultrasound guidance.

The advantages of the Mammotome system over traditional core biopsies are:
- A greater tissue sample is produced, which allows for a more precise diagnosis.
- The procedure is faster and less traumatic, as only 1 puncture is needed (as opposed to 4 or 5).
- The system inserts the needle without the release "shot" of the pistol-type mechanism.

The only disadvantage to this system is its high cost.

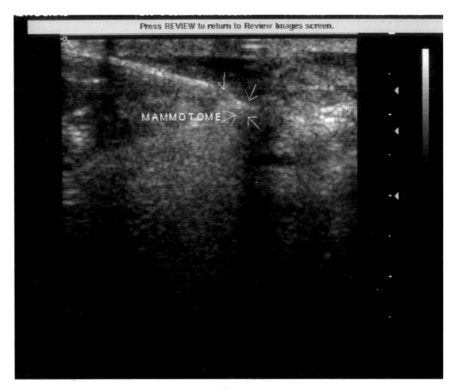

Mammotome needle within a lesion

Ductal Carcinoma *in situ*
Incidence

A) Clinical Diagnosis 1975-80	2-4% of palpable cancers
B) Mammographical Diagnosis (and screening campaigns) 1980-95	15-20% of cancers
C) Current Day (screening campaigns and US technology)	22 to 45% of cancers

Dershaw. Cardeñosa G. 1997

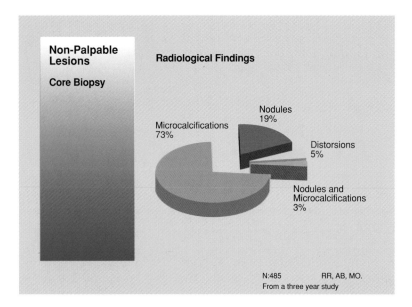

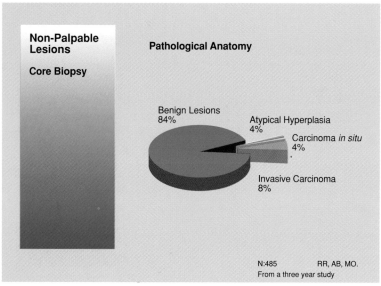

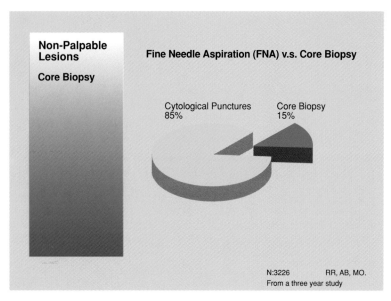

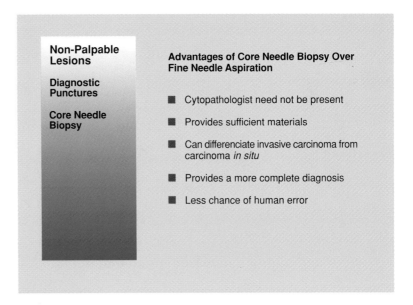

Non-Palpable Lesions

Diagnostic Punctures

Core Needle Biopsy

Advantages of Core Needle Biopsy Over Fine Needle Aspiration

- Cytopathologist need not be present
- Provides sufficient materials
- Can differenciate invasive carcinoma from carcinoma *in situ*
- Provides a more complete diagnosis
- Less chance of human error

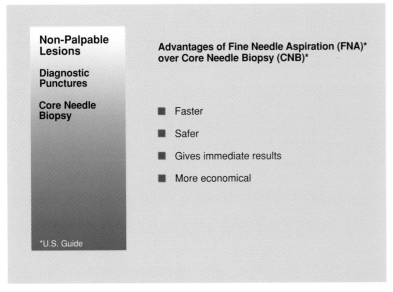

Non-Palpable Lesions

Diagnostic Punctures

Core Needle Biopsy

Advantages of Fine Needle Aspiration (FNA)* over Core Needle Biopsy (CNB)*

- Faster
- Safer
- Gives immediate results
- More economical

*U.S. Guide

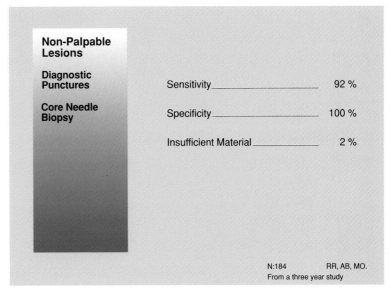

Non-Palpable Lesions

Diagnostic Punctures

Core Needle Biopsy

Sensitivity	92 %
Specificity	100 %
Insufficient Material	2 %

N:184   RR, AB, MO.
From a three year study

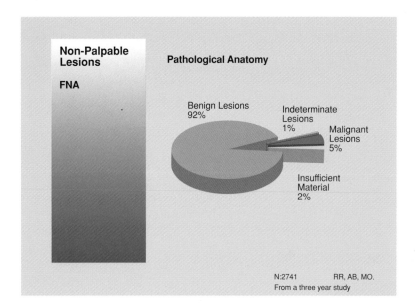

Non-Palpable Lesions

FNA

Pathological Anatomy

Benign Lesions 92%

Indeterminate Lesions 1%

Malignant Lesions 5%

Insufficient Material 2%

N:2741   RR, AB, MO.
From a three year study

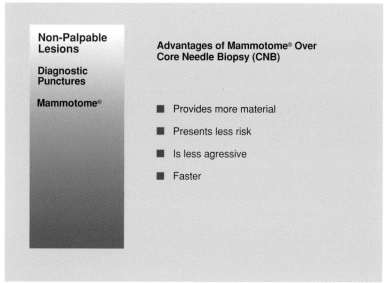

Non-Palpable Lesions

Diagnostic Punctures

Mammotome®

Advantages of Mammotome® Over Core Needle Biopsy (CNB)

■ Provides more material

■ Presents less risk

■ Is less agressive

■ Faster

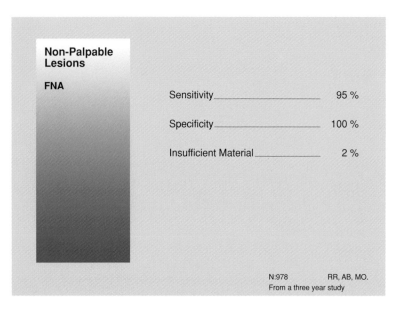

Non-Palpable Lesions

FNA

Sensitivity _____ 95 %

Specificity _____ 100 %

Insufficient Material _____ 2 %

N:978   RR, AB, MO.
From a three year study

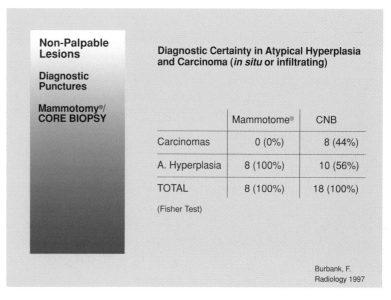

Non-Palpable Lesions

Diagnostic Punctures

Mammotomy®/ CORE BIOPSY

Diagnostic Certainty in Atypical Hyperplasia and Carcinoma (*in situ* or infiltrating)

	Mammotome®	CNB
Carcinomas	0 (0%)	8 (44%)
A. Hyperplasia	8 (100%)	10 (56%)
TOTAL	8 (100%)	18 (100%)

(Fisher Test)

Burbank, F.
Radiology 1997

Non-Palpable Lesions

Diagnostic Punctures

Mammotomy®/ CORE BIOPSY

Diagnostic Certainty in Ductal Carcinomas

	Mammotome®	CNB
In situ	32 (100%)	46 (84%)
Infiltrating		9 (16%)
TOTAL	32 (100%)	55 (100%)

(Fisher Test)

Burbank, F.
Radiology 1997 202: 843-847

Non-Palpable Lesions

Diagnostic Punctures

FNA

Sensitivity _____ 68 -100%

Specificity _____ 82 -100%

Insufficient Material _____ 2 - 36%

213

References

- Kline, T. S. et al. Guides to Clinical Aspiratorion Biopsy: Breast. Igaku-Shoin, New York, 1989.
- D'Orsi C. J. et al. Interventional Breast Ultrasonography. Semin Ultrasound CT MR 1989; 10:132-138.
- Fornage, B. D. Interventional Ultrasound of the Breast. En McGahan J. P. (ed.): Interventional Ultrasound. Williams & Wilkins, Baltimore, 1990; 71-83.
- Fornage, B. D. et al. Ultrasound-guided. Needle Biopsy of the Breast and Other Interventional Procedures. *Radiology* Clinic of North America 1992; 30:167-185.
- Hopper, K. D. et al. Aumated Biopsy Decives: A Blinded Evaluation. *Radiology* 187:653-660, 1993.
- Tabar, L. et al. Percutaneous Breast Biopsy. New York, Raven Press, 1993, p. Xi.
- Liberman L.et al. Radiography of Microcalcifications in Stereotaxic Mammary Core Biopsy Specimens. *Radiology* 190:223-225, 1994.
- Brenner, R. J. et al. Percutaneous Core Biopsy of the Breast: a Multisite Prospective Trial, abstracted. *Radiology* 1994; 193(P): 295.
- Parker S., Burbank, F. Radiology 1996; 200:11-20
- Burbank, F. Radiology 1996; 202:843-847

12

Artifacts and Errors

M. E. Lanfranchi

Unlike other human anatomical structures whose echogenic patterns change very little, the breast is a dynamic organ which undergoes changes during the entire menstrual cycle due to the influence of hormones. Pregnancy and age also cause changes in the breast, and thus extensive specialized training is required to prevent errors.

It is also very important that mammary examinations be conducted in the following order:

- **Patient history and antecedents.**
- **Inspection and palpation.**
- **Mammographical examination.**
- **Ultrasound examination.**

Examinations should always be carried out in this order, because the same image may be interpreted in different ways according to the patient's history, antecedents, and/or mammographical results.

The following are a few examples:

1. Hypoechoic mass with heterogeneous echostructure; predominantly solid and with irregular borders.
May be:
- Carcinoma
- Hematoma
- Post-surgical granuloma

2. Hypoechoic mass with significant sonic attenuation.
May be:
- Carcinoma
- Calcified fibroadenoma
- Fat necrosis

3. Image with sonic attenuation
May be:
- Scar tissue
- Fibrosis
- Cooper's ligament
- Calcification
- Ribs

Because of the possible ambiguity of some ultrasound images it is important that a combined diagnosis be performed if any breast anomaly is discovered. Ultrasound has resolution limitations and is not appropiate for the diagnosis of microcalcifications which are not located in a nodule. However, the combination of mammography and ultrasound provides the most complete diagnosis.

Most errors are due to the following factors:
- Inadequate equipment.
- Improper setting of the equipment controls.
- Pseudonodular adipose infiltration in the parenchyma.
- Cooper's ligaments.
- Cartilage and rib borders.
- Exploration of the nipple with inadequate compression.
- Cysts with the interior echoes (reverberation or real echoes).
- Fibroadenoma (resembling carcinoma or with calcified areas).
- Carcinomas with a diameter of less than 1 cm (which may appear benign in 20% of cases. See Chapter 5).
- Linear images within a silicone implant (do not confuse folding with intracapsular rupture. See Chapter 9).

Obviously, the chance of error also depends upon:

- **The ultrasound operator's training and experience.**
- **The quality of the equipment used.**
- **Adequate study of previous mammographies.**

If the ultrasound image produced is unsatisfactory one can try changing the position of the transducer, changing the position of the patient, rotating the transducer along a horizontal plane, adjusting the pressure of the transducer on the tissues, and finally (but not least importantly) adjusting the controls of the equipment.

If the power gain is not adjusted correctly an image of a cyst may appear solid and to have interior echoes (see figs. 12.1 and 12.2).

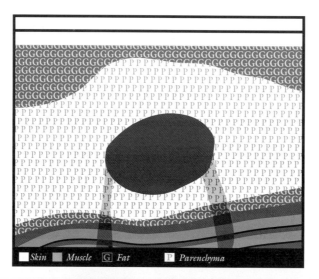

Skin ▪ Muscle G Fat P Parenchyma

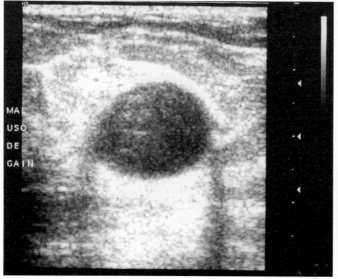

Figure. 12.1 Image demonstrating improper use of the grey-scale gain; lack of contrast is produced by adjusting too far into the white scale. The nodule appears with fine interior echoes and the other layers produce too many echoes.

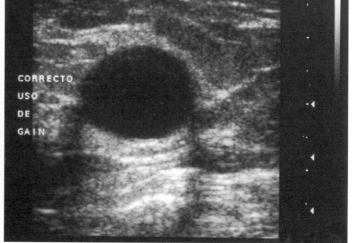

Figure. 12.2 Correct use of the grey scale gain on the same breast as Figure. 12.1 produces an image of a liquid-filled anechoic nodule with smooth borders, enhanced echoes in the posterior wall and lateral sonic attenuation.

An artifact is an anomaly in the ultrasound image which does not correspond to a reflective structure and can lead to diagnostic error. An example of this is reverberation, or the multiple reflection phenomenon, which is caused by numerous reflections between the transducer and the tissues. Acoustic impedance causes a large percentage of the sound to be bounced back and forth between the transducer and the tissues.

Artifacts appear as lines or groups of echoes of decreasing intensity. In order to avoid this phenomenon one should change either the angle of exploration or the frequency of the transducer, or both.

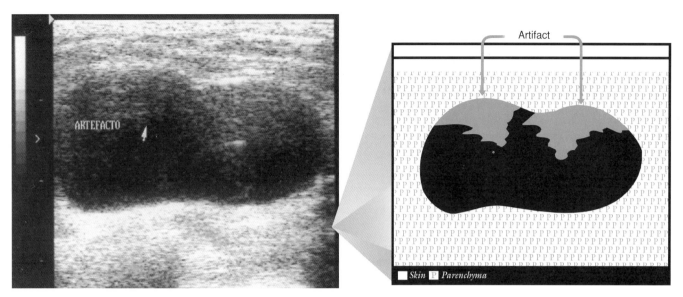

Figure. 12.3 Image of a nodule with smooth and regular borders and enhanced echoes on the posterior wall; beneath the anterior wall there is a band of fine echoes produced by reverberation or multiple reflection phenomenon.

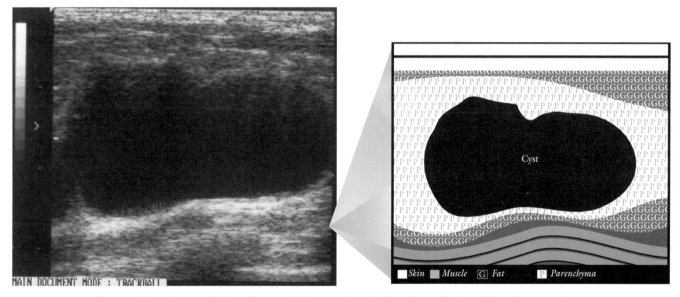

Figure. 12.4 Same nodule as Figure. 12.3; reverberation has been eliminated by adjusting the power gain of the grey scale and modifying the angle of the ultrasound beam.

If hypoechoic images appear within an echogenic parenchyma one should determine whether the images correspond to actual nodules or pseudonodular zones of fatty infiltration. This can be done by rotating the transducer in order to investigate the connections the image may have with neighboring adipose areas.

When an ultrasound beam strikes a structure of high acoustic impedance (such as calcium or bone) no echoes will be produced in the area directly behind the structure. This is called a "sonic shadow" and the higher the frequency of the transducer the more pronounced it will be. Sonic shadows are not uncommon when the ultrasound beam strikes the Cooper's ligaments at certain angles, and should not be mistaken for a pathology.

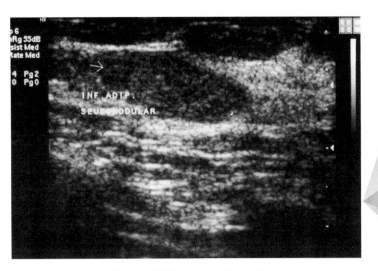
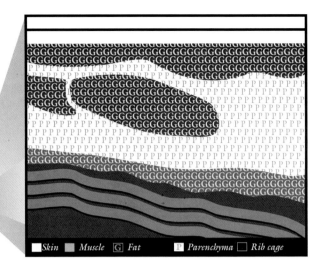

Figure. 12.5 Image of two hypoechoic pseudonodular images within mammary parenchyma which produce the same level of echogenicity as adipose tissue. This image is of fatty infiltration and not nodules, so the form and appearance of the images changes significantly as the transducer is moved.

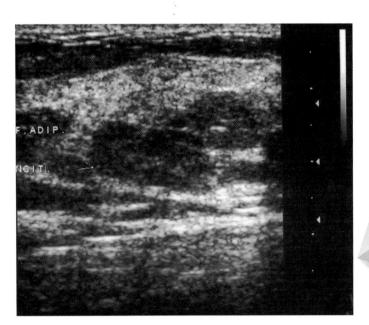
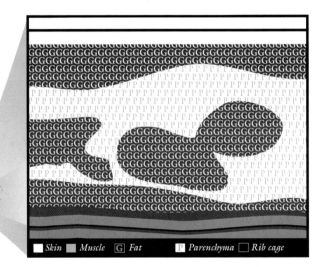

Figure. 12.6 A case similar to that of Figure. 12.5. The image clears when the angle of the ultrasound beam is adjusted.

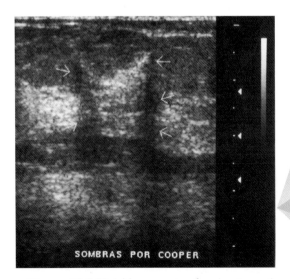
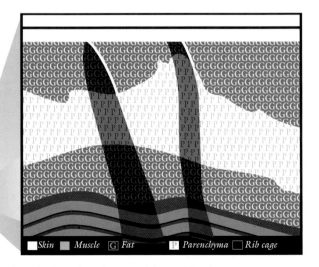

Figure. 12.7 Variable amounts of sonic attenuation are produced when the ultrasound beam hits the Cooper's ligaments. This is corrected by exploring other layers.

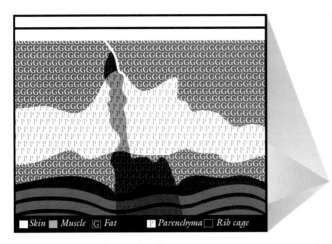

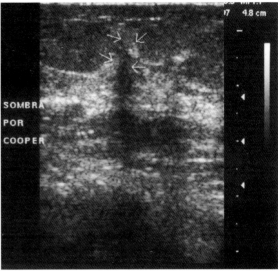

Figure. 12.8 Cooper's ligaments may produce sonic attenuation when the ultrasound beam passes through the breast; this attenuation should not be mistaken for a pathology.

When the ultrasound beam falls upon the border of a rib the image produced may show significant sonic attenuation behind the rib itself, which may or may not allow one to distinguish the shape of the structure. Again, this should not be mistaken for a nodular pathology.

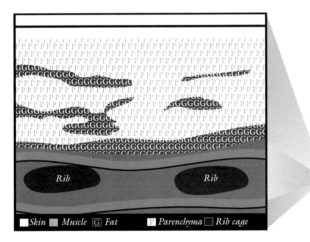

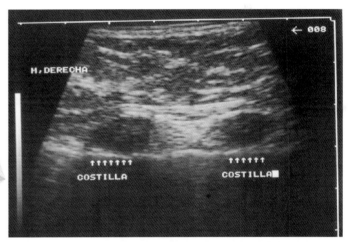

Figure. 12.9 This view of the breast includes the skin and descends to the ribcage. The two nodular images located deep within the breast are actually ribs, which becomes more obvious when the transducer is turned.

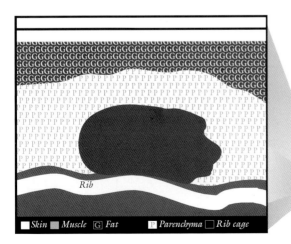

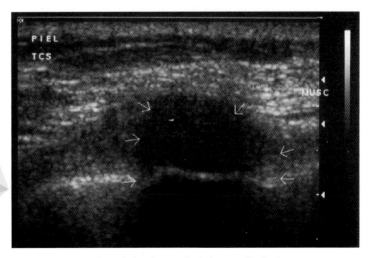

Figure. 12.10 Another image of a rib, which appears as a pseudonodular, hypoechoic image displaying very low echogenicity.

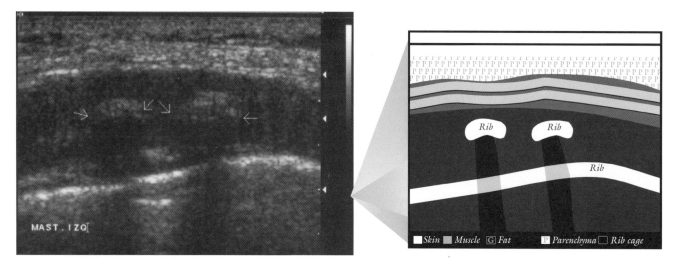

Figure. 12.11 Two ribs within thinned parenchyma which appear as half-moon shaped hyperechogenic images with posterior sonic attenuation due to the ultrasound beam striking the anterior rib border.

Two situations may arise in ultrasound examination of the retroaerolar region:

1) If the nipple is flattened while performing the examination it may project a shadow which appears to be a nodule deep in the tissues.

2. Inadequate compression of the tissues may produce an image with shadows and distortions in the tissue layers.

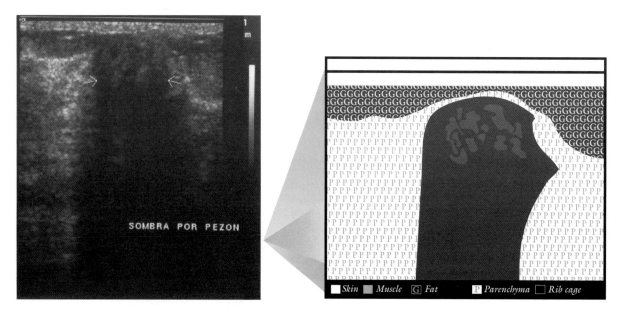

Figure. 12.12 When the transducer is placed directly above the nipple significant sonic attenuation may occur which obscures the anatomical layers below.

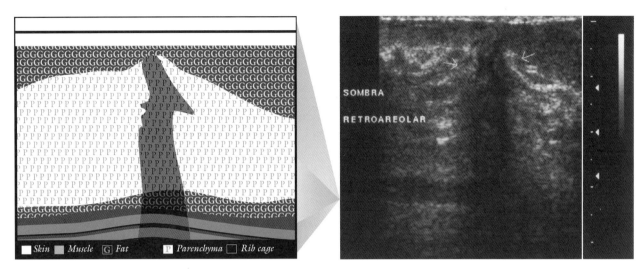

Figure. 12.13 This image shows the same placement of the transducer as in Figure. 12.12; the image can be greatly improved by modifying the pressure exerted on the breast.

Sequelae in patients who have had previous surgery should be differentiated from possible simultaneous pathologies, or recurrence of carcinomas.

Sonic attenuation may be produced if the surgical scar is complicated by fibrosis.

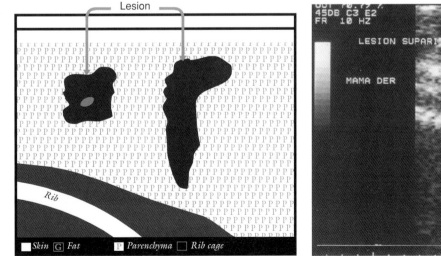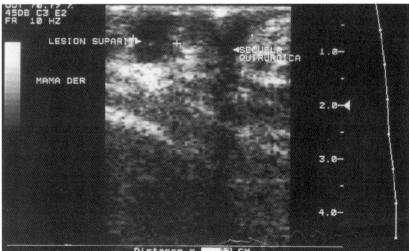

Figure. 12.14 Image of two hypoechoic nodules; the one on the right displays sonic attenuation and is a scar sequela complicated with fibrosis resulting from previous surgery for a carcinoma. The nodule on the right is a focus of cancer due to a possible local recurrence.

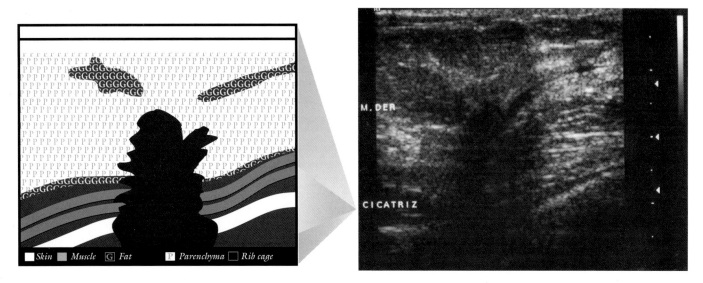

Figure. 12.15 Image of a surgical scar with fibrosis in a patient who had undergone surgery to remove a benign breast nodule. The fibrosis produces significant sonic attenuation, as seen in the center of the image.

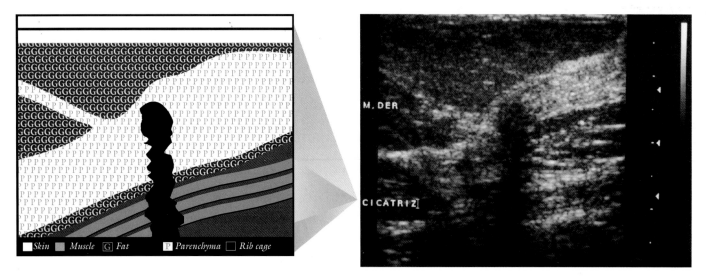

Figure. 12.16 Another image of sonic attenuation produced by post-surgical fibrosis.

As stated in previous chapters, there are reliable signs by which one can differentiate a solid benign nodule from a malignant nodule.

However, in cases of poorly-defined images there may be some doubt. Figure 12.17 shows just such a case, in which a solid homogeneous nodule with irregular borders suspected of atypia was diagnosed by biopsy as fibroadenoma.

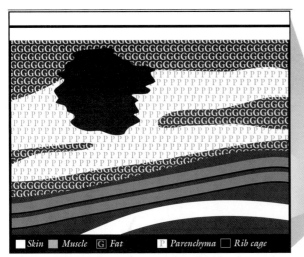

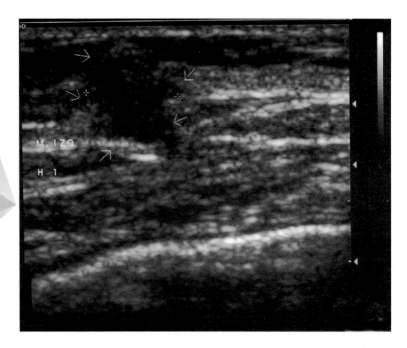

Figure. 12.17 Image of a solid, palpable, hypoechoic nodule close to the skin with irregular borders. The borders would indicate a carcinoma, but a biopsy confirmed this to be a case of fibroadenoma.

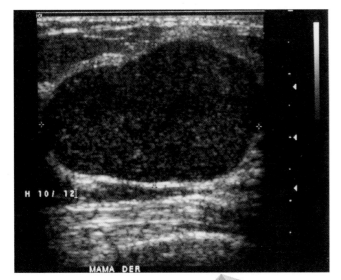

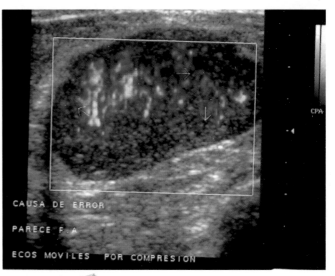

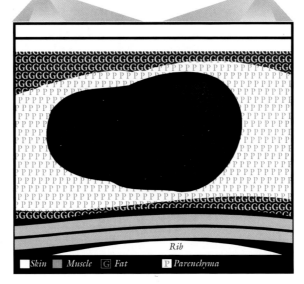

Figure. 12.18 Image of a hypoechoic nodule with defined borders which appears to be a fibroadenoma. However, during the evaluation the fine interior echoes moved to the posterior wall, a movement detected with power Doppler. Diagnostic puncture confirmed a cystic dilation with galactophoritis.

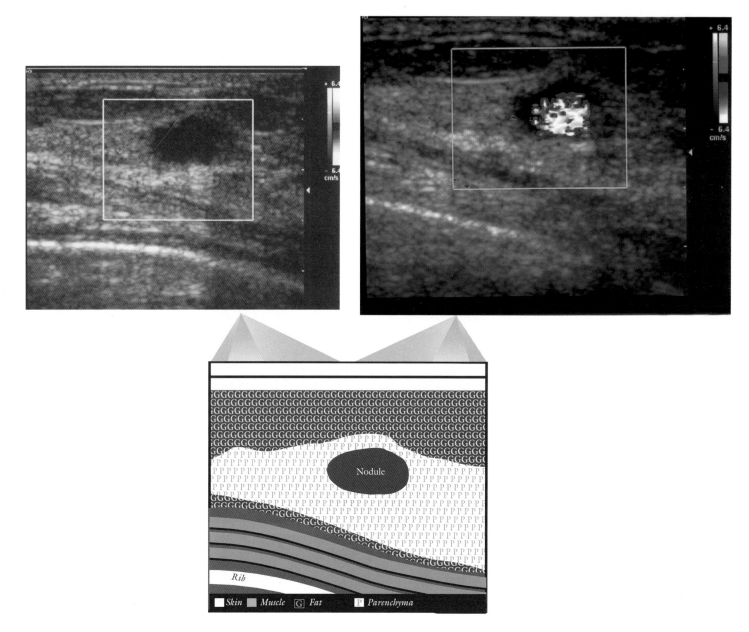

Figure. 12.19 Image of an anechoic, non-palpable nodule 8mm in size which was diagnosed as a simple cyst. The image on the right displays the incorrect use of the power gain, it is set to 100% and produces an artifact within the cyst. This is corrected by adjusting the gain to 80%.

On the other hand, some calcified fibroadenomas may appear to be carcinomas if they are not examined by mammography.

In summary, an ultrasound examination should include a detailed study of the image in order to eliminate artifacts and errors and to arrive at a diagnosis compatible with a certain pathology. This diagnosis should be correlated with clinical and mammographical examinations, in order to reach a conclusion which takes into consideration all signs and symptoms.

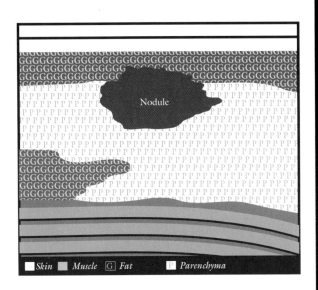

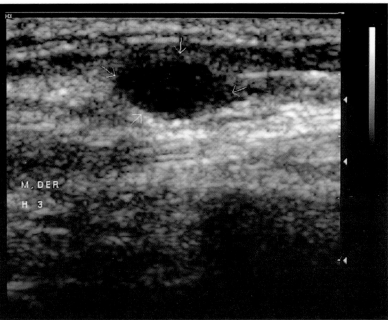

Figs. 12.20.1., 12.20.2 Images of a solid, elongated nodule with clean borders in one sector and irregularities in another, and a vascular signal picked up by Color Doppler which could indicate either a fibroadenoma or a carcinoma. The nodule was confirmed to be a fibroadenoma.

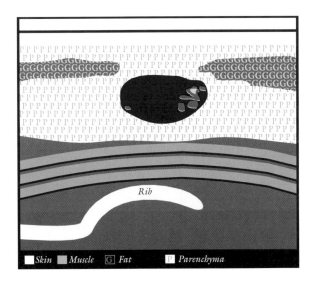

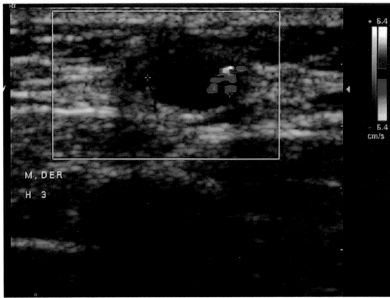

13

Ultrasound in Post-Menopausal Women

M. E. Lanfranchi

Introduction

In the post-menopausal period the mammary gland demonstrates a reduction in cell size and a breakdown of the ducts and alveoli, conditions frequently associated with cysts and metaplasia. Alterations found in this stage may also be sequelae from pathologies treated previously.

Images of post-menopausal breasts show fatty infiltration which gradually replaces the parenchyma. This is an advantage in mammography because most nodules and lesions contrast well with the resultant radiolucent background. However, the opposite is true with ultrasound, as one is generally searching for hypoechoic lesions in a breast which has become hypoechoic itself.

Common Pathologies

Calcifications appear frequently in the post-menopausal breast and may be due to various pathologies (for this reason it is important to determine if the calcifications are glandular, ductal, or vascular in nature). Due to the limitations of ultrasound, microcalcifications are normally located by mammography and then correlated with an ultrasound study.

According to a study by Bernardello et al. 20% of biopsies performed on post-menopausal women with non-palpable lesions revealed microcalcifications and opacities, and in the same group one case of benign breast disease was found for every 14 cancers.

According to a study published by Dixon ductal ectasia appears most frequently between 40 and 50 years of age. This pathology is easily diagnosed with the proper equipment, it results in the dilation of the ducts, generally accompanied by lobular atrophy and fibrosis and lipomatosis of the stroma. Ductal ectasia accounts for approximately 3% of all benign breast diseases and can be temporary or chronic.

The symptoms associated with ductal ectasia are

- **Discharge.**
- **Umbilicated or retracted nipple.**
- **Eczema or irritation of the nipple caused by secretion.**

Diagnosis is greatly facilitated by consideration of the patient's medical history before the physical and ultrasound examinations. Pathologies which produce similar symptoms (such as papillary tumors) should also be ruled out.

227

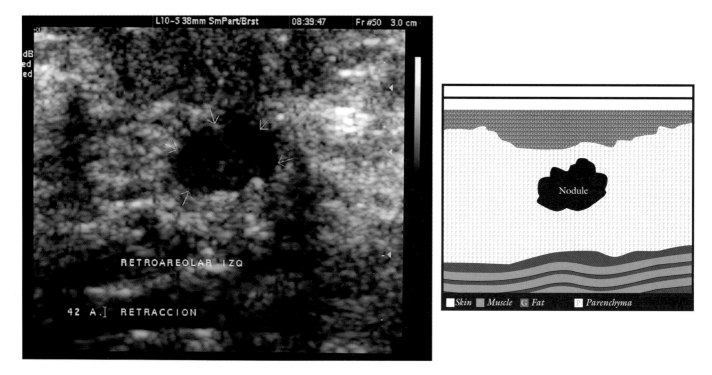

Fig. 13.1 Image of a solid nodule at the retroareolar level in a 42 year-old patient complaining of nipple retraction who had undergone menopause 4 years ago. The nodule displays low echogenicity, irregular borders, and spicules. A biopsy confirmed a papillary tumor, which was removed by conservative resection.

Ductal ectasia may provoke secretions which build up in the breast causing inflammation and/or infection, and can lead to galactophoritis.

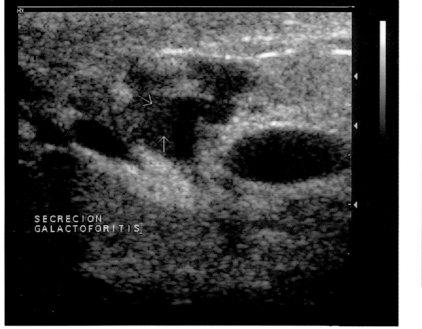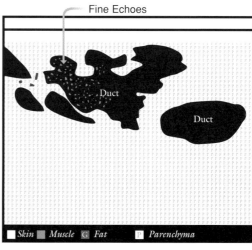

Fig. 13.2 Image of lactiferous ducts affected by galactophoritis in a 41 year-old patient who complained of spontaneous secretion from the nipple. The image shows affected ducts which have irregular borders and varying diameters.

Infectious processes may be found in older women as a result of the weakening of the immune system, or from diseases such as diabetes. These processes may involve the nipple and/or the skin of the breast.

The diverse group of pathologies referred to as "dysplasia" can be divided into two basic types: **involutive fibrocystic disease** and **proliferative fibrocystic disease**. Images of these pathologies appear in Chapter 6.

In older women it is common to encounter traumas of various degrees of severity caused by falls, from simple contusions which are difficult to detect with ultrasound to collections of fluid and blood (liquid or coagulated) which are much easier to detect.

Fat necrosis can be caused by trauma (either direct or post-surgical; see Chapter 10) and after a period of time it may appear in ultrasound as a hypoechoic nodular image, which makes it necessary to differentiate from a carcinoma.

Surgical scars should be closely examined, especially if the patient has suffered neoplasia in the past.

According to a study conducted by Devitt calcified fibroadenomas may be found in between 1 and 4% of post-menopausal women.

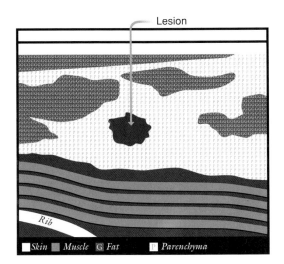

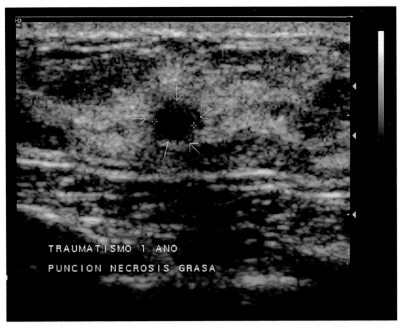

Fig. 13.3 Image of fat necrosis in a patient with an antecedent trauma one year prior. In the center of the parenchyma appears a hypoechoic image 4mm in size with irregular and partially defined borders.

The extent of calcification is variable and depends upon the age of the nodule.

When these nodules reach a certain volume they can cause significant sonic attenuation and force one to carry out a differential diagnosis with a carcinoma (this should be done by mammography; see Chapter 4).

Phyllodes tumors are rare in older women, but when they do appear they tend to be large, benign, and slow to develop.

Pathologies Affecting Post-Menopausal Women:

Most Frequent:	Fibrocystic Disease
	Fibroadenoma
Least Frequent:	Proliferative Dysplasia
	Phyllodes Tumors
	Papillary Tumors
	Lipomas

Post-Menopausal Breast Carcinoma

According to the American Cancer Society, breast cancer rates are as follows for the age groups listed:

40 to 49 years:	**18.6%**
50 to 59 years:	**15.6%**
60 to 69 years:	**22.7%**
70 to 79 years:	**24.3%**
80 years or more:	**13.9%**

According to this information cancers are most frequent in women between 70 and 79 years of age. These cancers range in histological types from microcalcifications to nodules, and may have any of the characteristics described in Chapter 5. Generally, cancers grow slowly in older women, but unfortunately many cancers are in advanced stages when they are diagnosed because many older women are unaware of self-examination techniques or because the cancer produces no pain.

14

Color Doppler and Related Technologies

M. E. Lanfranchi

Introduction

"Doppler" is the last name of Austrian physicist Christian Johann Doppler. Doppler was studying phenomena produced by the effects of light, and arrived at a theory in 1842 which would later aid in the development of ultrasound technologies.

More than one hundred years later, in 1955, Shigeo Samotura, a physicist at the University of Osaka designed a device which allowed the tracking of blood flow through the veins and arteries.

In 1974 the duplex system was developed which combined a two-dimensional ultrasound image with the Doppler system. This advance allowed doctors to study extremely small or difficult to reach areas (e.g. the interior of an artery).

Until 1996 the Doppler system used a continuous operating mode in which the transducer consisted of two crystals, one which emitted ultrasound, and another which received the signal representing the movement of blood. This was replaced by a pulsed Doppler system which uses one crystal for emission and reception, allowing one to select the depth of ultrasound penetration for greater precision.

Certain researchers of mammary pathologies suggested the possibility of conducting a vascular analysis using the continuous system, but the two-dimensional system proved superior because of the vast improvement it provided in the quality of the grey scale.

A number of authors have published articles analyzing the physical characteristics of the Doppler system and describing the appearance of benign and malignant breast pathologies in Doppler images.

Doppler technology continues to advance, especially in the area of color Doppler systems. The color Doppler system combines Doppler duplex with a vascular signal in color. Triplex mode, a combination of imaging, color, and spectral Doppler is capable of collecting and displaying data in 'real time'.

Blood flow is codified and applied to the ultrasound image by the color Doppler system; blood movement is represented by various colors ranging from white or yellow to blue. A color map (color assignment, color coding) assigns these colors to various velocities. The range of velocities which can be displayed is adjusted by the use of the Pulse Repitition Frequency (PRF) controls. Slow blood flows can be detected by adjusting the PRF to a low setting (however, doing so may produce aliasing).

The specific area where the color Doppler imaging takes place, referred to as the color box (or color region of interest, ROI) is also selected and controlled by the Doppler operator. In addition to qualitative information on blood flow, color Doppler provides quantitative information such as the resistance index, systole/diastole (S-D) ratio, acceleration, etc.

The variance map is a display which uses different color hues to provide information concerning the estimated variance of the Doppler signal. The color maps of color Doppler machines generally vary according to manufacturer, but red is normally used for values above the baseline and blue for colors below it.

The angle of incidence is an important factor in both color and spectral Doppler. If an angle of 90° is used, no vascular signal will appear (however, a black area appears when using color Doppler). Research has shown that in order to obtain a clear signal the angle of incidence should be less than 60°. The ideal angle is 0°, but this angle may not necessarily provide the most information.

The problems associated with incidence angles and vascular tortuosity were addressed by the development of the amplitude map for color Doppler, which has been manufactured under names such as "Power", Angio", "Amplitude Imaging", etc. The colors of the amplitude map do not represent blood flow velocities, but rather correspond to the amplitude of the Doppler signal itself. Similarly, Doppler in power mode (and the corresponding power map) shows colors which represent the power of the Doppler signal, instead of its frequency. Doppler used in this manner is capable of detecting very slow blood flows. In fact, some manufacturers state that Doppler in power mode is 3-4 times as sensitive to slow blood flows as Doppler which measures frequency.

Advantages and Limitations of Color Doppler

Advantages
- Allows evaluation of the blood flow.
- Allows rapid identification of the vascular structure.
- Allows a quantitative measure of velocity.
- Sensitivity is adequate for vessels up to 1 mm thick.

Limitations
- Gives less spatial information, because only the vessels within the color box are colored.
- "Mode B" decreases definition.
- Can only be used at specific angles.
- Requires a skilled operator.

Advantages and Limitations of Amplitude/Energy Doppler

Advantages
- Can be used at any angle.
- Does not produce aliasing.
- Higher sensitivity:
  a) Allows deeper penetration.
  b) Detects smaller vessels.
  c) Detects slower flows.

Limitations
- Does not give information about direction of blood flow.
- Does not give information about flow velocity.
- Does not give information about the characteristics of the flow.

Color Doppler provides various types of information:

1) **If a vessel is visible, its location and the direction of flow can be determined.**

2) **The characteristics of the blood flow within the vessels can be determined.**

All flow characteristics are measured by the flow rate, either arterial or venous.

The indexes and velocities which can be measured are:
- **Systole/diastole index.**
- **The Pulse index** (P.I.; measured in cycles/second)
- **The Resistance index** (R.I.; indicates the resistance caused by blood flow through the vessel).

The velocities which can be analyzed are:
- **Systolic velocity** (S.V.)
- **Maximum systolic velocity** (M.S.V.)
- **Diastolic velocity** (D.V.)
- **End of diastole velocity** (E.D.V.)

These indexes and velocites allow for a thorough study of the characteristics of a given vessel.

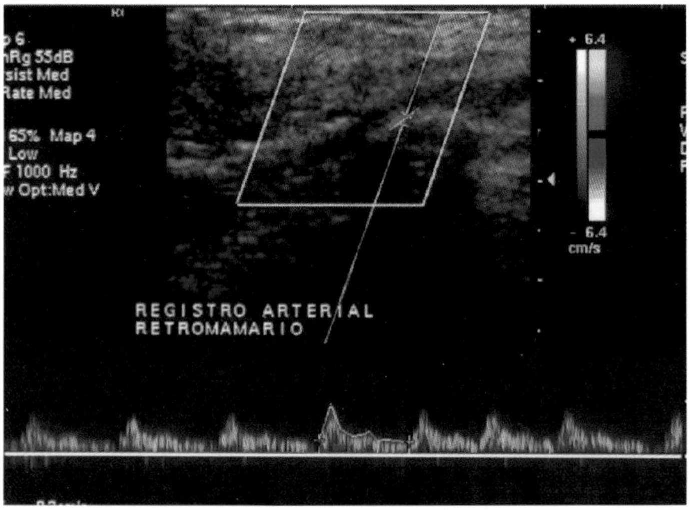

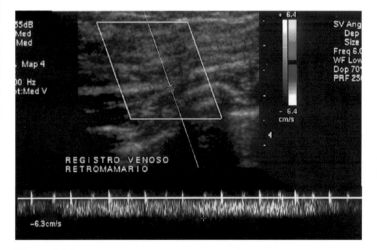

Figure 14.1.

Figure 14.2.

The arterial wave, like the cardiac cycle, consists of systolic and diastolic phases and shows pulsation. The venous wave has only one continuous cycle, does not show pulsation, and varies only with the respiratory cycle.

The Doppler System in Breast Evaluations

The various Doppler systems allow the evaluation of both the internal and external mammary arteries and the perforating branches. More importantly, Doppler can detect neovascularization present in breast tumors.

Neoangiogenic vessels are characterized by their lack of a muscle layer (see fig. 14.3).

Vessels

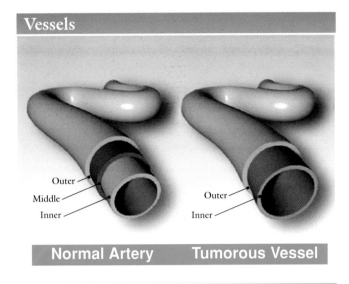

Outer
Middle
Inner

Outer
Inner

Normal Artery   **Tumorous Vessel**

Figure 14.3

Tumor Growth Linked to Angiogenesis

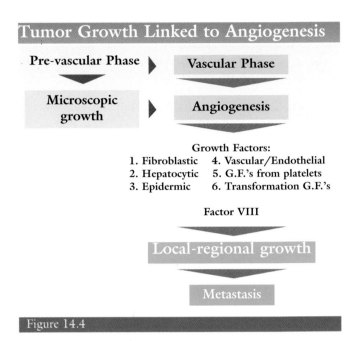

Pre-vascular Phase ► Vascular Phase

Microscopic growth ► Angiogenesis

Growth Factors:
1. Fibroblastic   4. Vascular/Endothelial
2. Hepatocytic   5. G.F.'s from platelets
3. Epidermic   6. Transformation G.F.'s

Factor VIII

Local-regional growth

Metastasis

Figure 14.4

These vessels are approximately 0.5 mm in diameter. When tumor cells first begin to multiply there is a non-vascular stage, but once a volume of 10^6 is reached, vascular support becomes necessary and vessels are formed, allowing neoplastic cells to enter the blood stream. So, this vascular stage is characterized by rapid tumor growth, bleeding, and the potential for metastasis.

The secretion of collagenases and plasminogen-stimulating factors is responsible for the invasive and chemotactic behavior of tumor cells. Ultimately, in order to survive and reproduce in a metastatic environment neoplastic cells must induce angiogenesis. The most important and often-studied angiogenic factor is a member of the fibroblastic growth factor (FGF) family, but six other factors have been identified, each with different characteristics. How this factor is activated is still unknown, but it is studied with immunohistochemical techniques using monoclonal antibodies.

Active tumors may induce the secretion of high levels of FGF, which enters the blood stream and can be detected in urine. FGF levels in urine may be used to monitor a patient's progress or establish a prognosis.

In summary, the degree of neovascularization measured by histological studies of cancers correlates with the presence of metastasis. Architecturally, these vascular structures form intratumoral and peritumoral networks and are responsible for the survival of the tumor. For this reason color Doppler is extremely useful in the study of breast tumors.

Angiogenesis-Dependent Tumor Growth

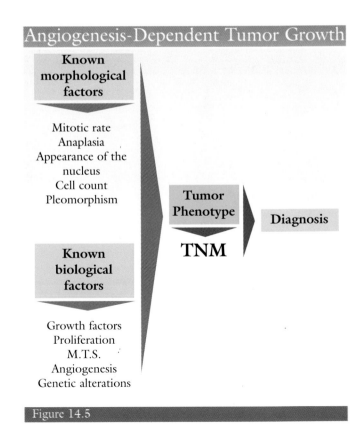

Known morphological factors

Mitotic rate
Anaplasia
Appearance of the nucleus
Cell count
Pleomorphism

Tumor Phenotype

TNM

Diagnosis

Known biological factors

Growth factors
Proliferation
M.T.S.
Angiogenesis
Genetic alterations

Figure 14.5

A differential diagnosis between a benign and a malignant tumor is possible by an analysis of the color signal and flow rate information provided by color Doppler:

1) *An analysis of the color signal examines:*

The location of the vessel with respect to the tumor:

- Peripheral
- Penetrating
- Intratumoral

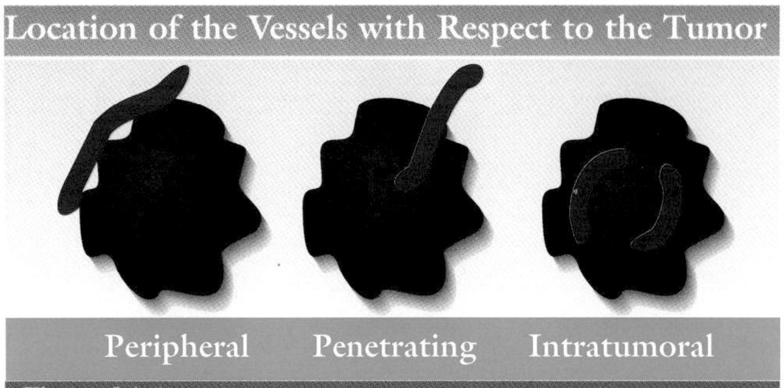

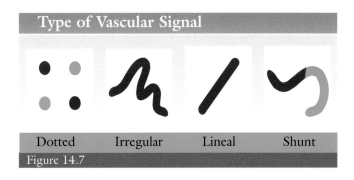

Figure 14.6

The number of vessels:

- Non-vascular
- Hypovascular (1 vessel)
- Vascular (2 or 3 vessels)
- Hypervascular (more than 5 vessels)

Type of vascular signal

- Dotted
- Irregular
- Lineal
- Shunt

Figure 14.7

This analysis is part of a quantitative-qualitative evaluation. The differences between benign and malignant tumors are listed on table 13.1

	Benign tumor	Malignant tumor
Number of vessels	None or few (*)	Multiple (*)
Vessels related to tumoral volume	1%	25% (*)
Intratumoral vessels	None (*)	5 or more (*)
Peripheric vessels	Scarce	Numerous
Tortuous vessels	Rare	Multiple
Shunts	Absent	Multiple

Table 13.1

(*) Some fibroadenomas, especially those larger than 20 or 25 mm in diameter, have multiple peripheral vessels.
(*) Small tumors (less than 1 cm), or those in older patients, may not present a vascular signal.

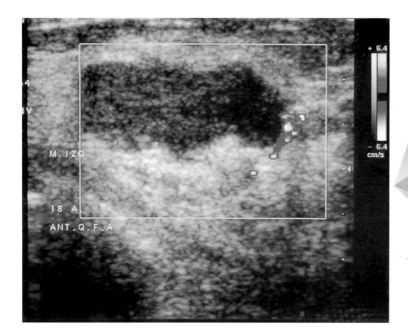

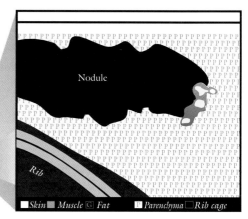

Fig. 14.8 Image of a fibroadenoma; it appears as a solid, lobulated nodule which produces a vascular signal on one of its borders.

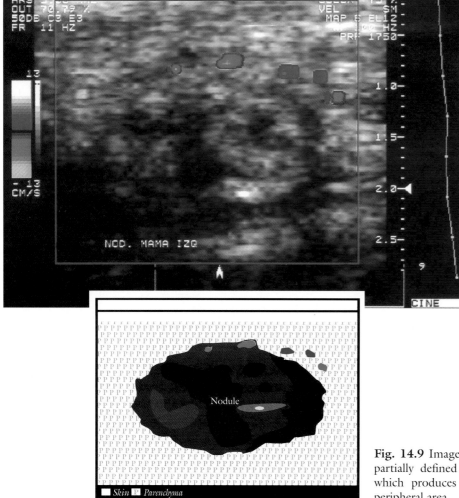

Fig. 14.9 Image of post-trauma fat necrosis; it appears as a partially defined heterogeneous mass 34 x 15mm in size which produces a color Doppler signal in the anterior-peripheral area.

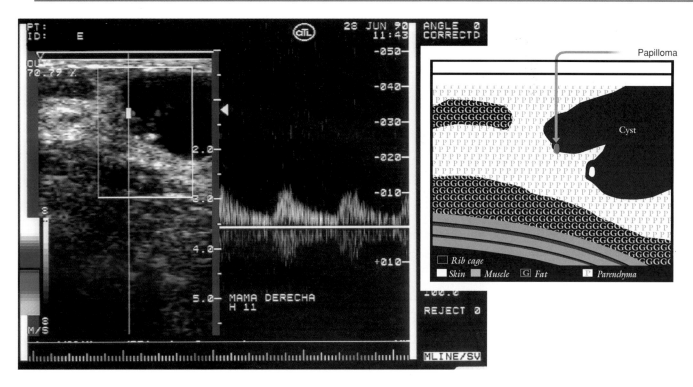

Fig. 14.10 Image of a cystic mass containing a small papilloma. A color Doppler signal is produced by a collection of blood vessels.

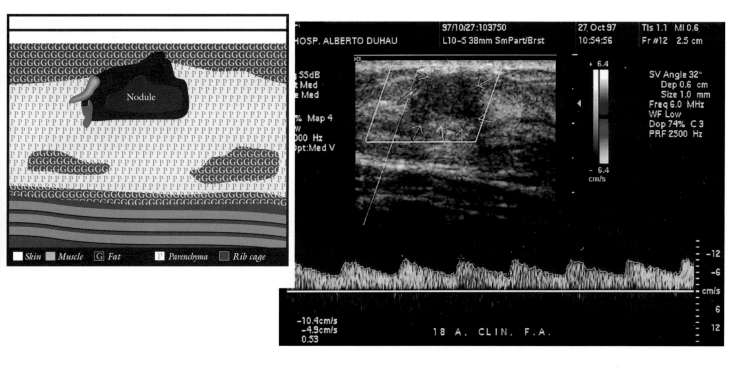

Fig. 14.11 Image of a solid, hypoechoic nodule with somewhat irregular borders in an 18 year-old patient. It was diagnosed by biopsy as a fibroadenoma. One signal was detected with color Doppler:

M.S.V.: 10.4 cm/s
D.V.: 4.9 cm/s
R.I.: 0.53

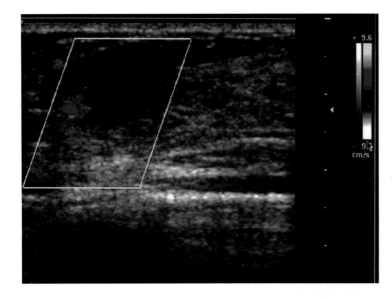

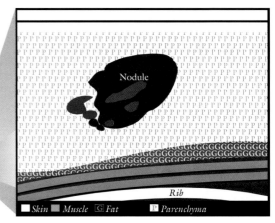

Fig. 14.12 Image of a solid nodule with lobulations and a vascular signal in one sector. It was diagnosed as a fibroadenoma.

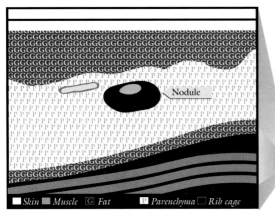

Fig. 14.13 Image of a solid nodule with a central area of greater echogenicity and one blood vessel located to the left of the nodule. Puncture revealed it to be an intramammary lymph node.

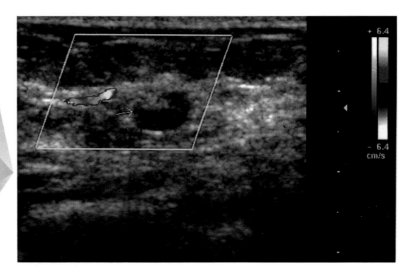

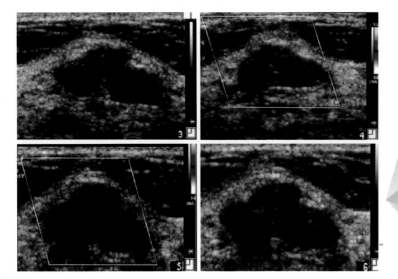

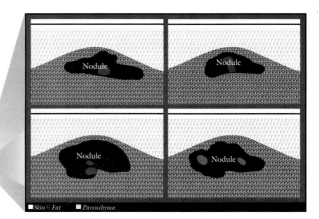

Fig. 14.14 Image of a solid, lobulated, palpable nodule which displays no vascular signal. It was diagnosed as a fibroadenoma.

While isolated peripheral vessels may be found in benign nodules, they are more common in malignant pathologies. In 92.5% of histologically confirmed carcinomas at least three vessels were found either within the tumor or penetrating it; 75% had 5 or more vessels similarly located.

Reasearch by E. Ueno et al. analyzes the relationship between the size and type of tumor (either benign or malignant) and the number of vessels it contains. According to their studies 18% of malignant tumors less than 10 mm in size had one vessel, while multiple vessels were found in 9.1% of the cases. 50% of tumors 20 mm or larger had multiple vessels.

On the other hand, 13.6% of benign tumors smaller than 10 mm had one vessel; 31.8% of those between 10 and 20 mm had one vessel, and 11.4% had more than two vessels.

Concerning the types of vessels found, irregular (or tortuous) vessels were found in 75% of malignant tumors and "dotted" vascular patterns were found in 78% of the cases. Irregular vessels were found in 14% of benign tumors, and "dotted" vascular patterns in 43% of the cases. Vessels may have either a central or a peripheral location in respect to the tumor. Centrally-located vessels in malignant tumors tend to have unevenly distributed and abnormal capillary proliferations, dilations, irregular diameters (from 50 to 500 millimicrons), and low pressure and resistance.

Peripherally-located penetrating vessels are usually accompanied by veins. Shunts may also be perhipherally-located, and usually cause an increased concentration of oxygen in the drainage veins, and a increase of the metabolism within the tumor.

Invasive Ductal Carcinoma

This carcinoma is distinguished by its growth rate and the amount of fibrous stroma it contains. There are two main types:

    1) Star-shaped or scirrhous carcinomas.
    2) Circumscribed carcinomas.

Scirrhous carcinomas display variable posterior sonic attenuation. They are hypovascular because the arteries are compressed by the surrounding tissues and blood flow within the tumor is low.

Circumscribed carcinomas (ductal carcinomas with a tubular papillary or solid tubular and medular hypercellular pattern) may display enhancement in the posterior wall and a pattern indicating an increase in vascularization.

A study of 50 carcinomas conducted by Rizzatto et al. using color Doppler showed flow signals in 90% of the cases and bi-directional flows in 93%. The flow signal was peripheral in 33.3% of the cases, central in 17.8%, and irregular in 48.9%. Average tumor size was 1.6 cm.

A semi-quantitative study based on the average number of vessels per square centimeter and the average color density of pixels has shown good results in the detection of vessels in malignant processes.

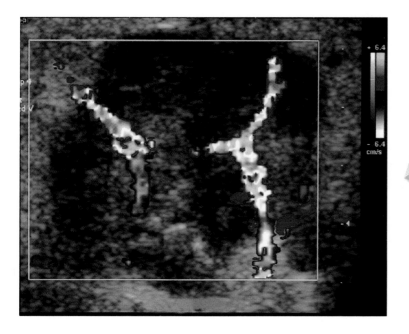

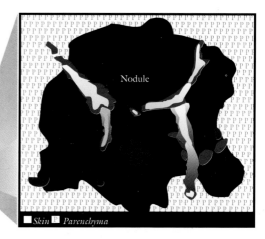

Fig. 14.15 Image of a solid, heterogeneous nodule displaying hypervascularization, It was diagnosed as a carcinoma.

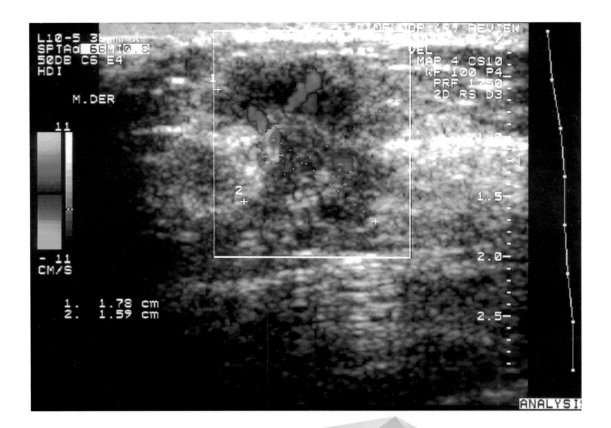

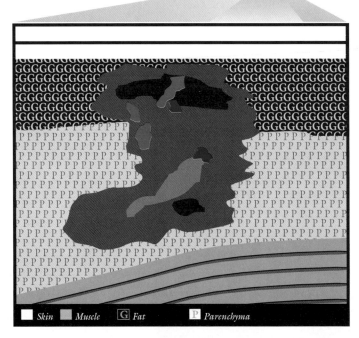

Skin   Muscle   G Fat   P Parenchyma

Fig. 14.16 Image of a solid nodule with irregular and poorly defined borders in some sectors. It produces heterogeneous echoes and five irregular color Doppler vascular signals. One of the vessels is tortuous. It was diagnosed as an infiltrating ductal carcinoma with a focus of necrosis.

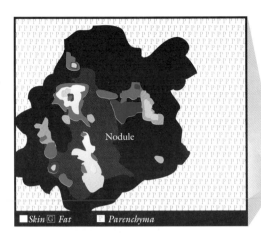

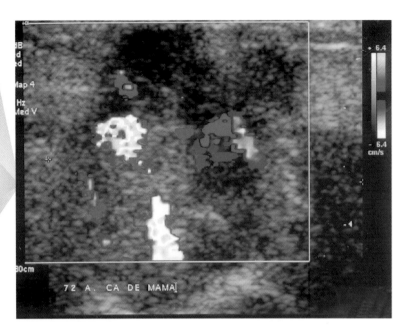

Fig. 14.17 Image of an infiltrating ductal carcinoma in a 72 year-old patient complaining of a painful, palpable nodule. Color Doppler shows a central area with increased vascularization.

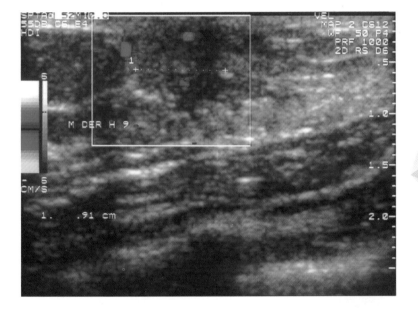

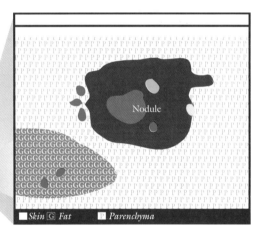

Figs. 14.18, 14.19 Images of a solid, heterogeneous nodule with irregular borders and a number of peripheral vascular signals. It was diagnosed as a carcinoma.

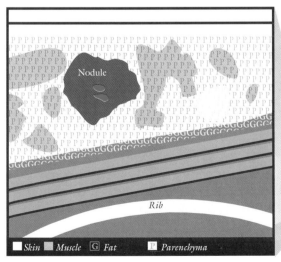

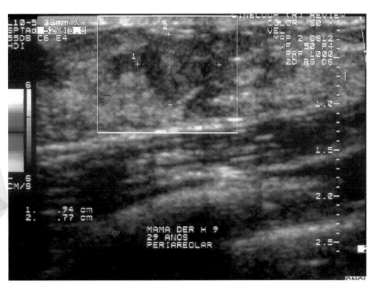

Fig. 14.19 See above.

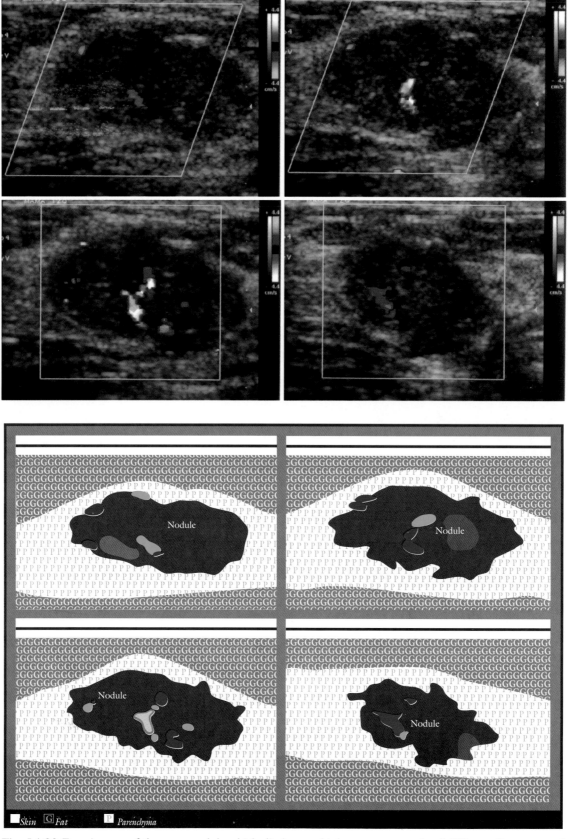

Fig. 14.20 Four images of the same nodule which displays multiple tortuous vessels of different diameters and lying in different directions. It was diagnosed as an infiltrating ductal carcinoma.

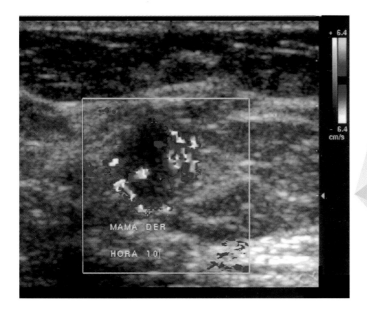

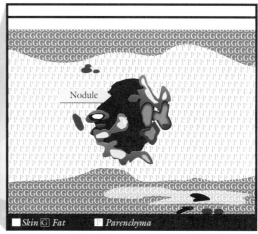

Fig. 14.21 Image of a solid, non-palpable nodule 10mm in diameter which displays intense central and peripheral vascularization with mosaicism. It was diagnosed as an infiltrating ductal carcinoma.

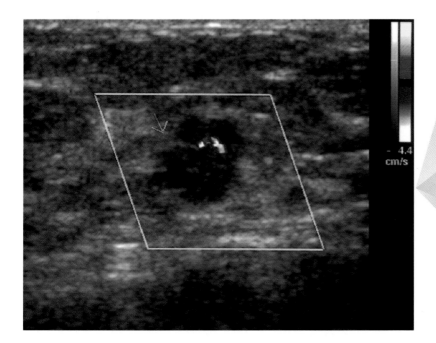

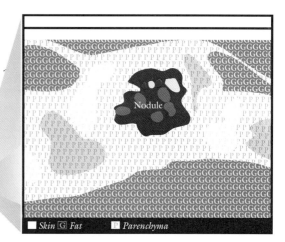

Figs. 14.22-14.24 Images of a solid, heterogeneous nodule with irregular borders and multiple internal and peripheral vessels. It was diagnosed as a carcinoma.

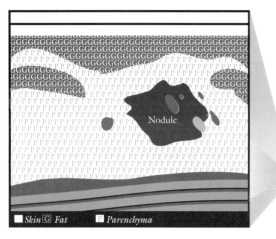

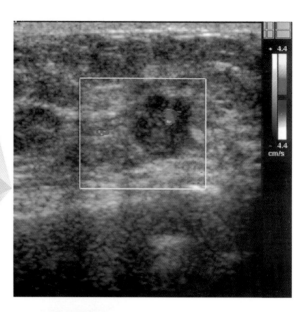

Fig. 14.23 See above.

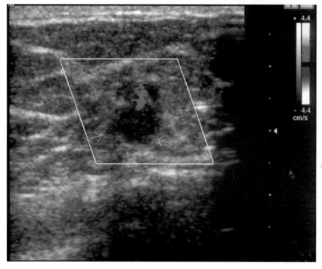

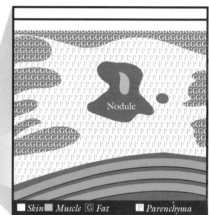

Fig. 14.24 See above.

Inflammatory and infectious diseases such as mastitis and abscesses may also result in an increase in the vascularization of the breast.

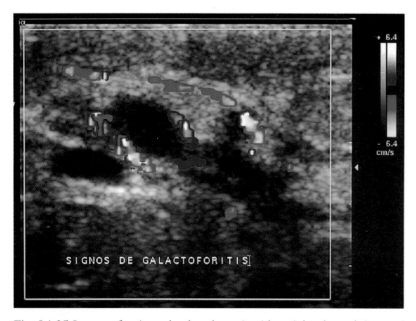

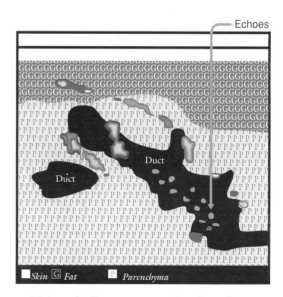

Fig. 14.25 Images of an irregular ductal ectasia with peripheral vessels in a patient complaining of yellow-green secretion from the nipple. Puncture confirmed a benign process.

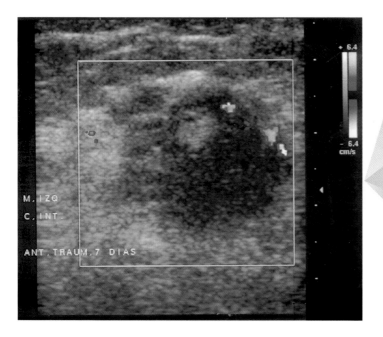

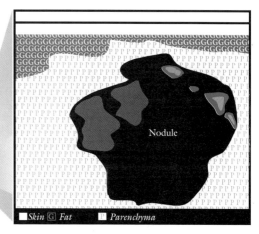

Fig. 14.26 Image of an organized hematoma in a patient with a trauma 7 days before; nodule is hypoechoic, heterogeneous, and has a peripheral vascular signal in one sector.

Recurrences of breast cancer display the same characteristics as the original tumor. Generally, malignant tumors are hypervascular, and have tortuous vessels and shunts. In some cases inability to locate a vascular signal may be due to improper use of the settings of the Doppler equipment (such as the wall filter or the pulse repetition filter). However, these problems are beyond the scope of this text and it is sufficient to note that the success of a study depends on proper technique and the proper use of the equipment.

Cosgrove et al. performed a study in which the percentage of vessels per cubic centimeter was calculated and compared to the percentage of color pixels. In a study published in 1993, 57 cancers out of 58 were detected; of these the percentage of vessels per cubic centimeter was 0.11 and these vessels occupied 1.76% of the area. Only 4% of the benign pathologies produced Doppler signals, and these were cases of fibroadenoma (which had an average of 0.06 vessels per cubic centimeter and occupied a small area less than 0.41%).

An investigation carried out by the author compared the following methods:
1) **Physical examination.**
2) **Mammography.**
3) **Ultrasound.**
4) **Color Doppler.**

The most successful methods were:
- **Ultrasound (96%)**
- **Color Doppler (92%)**

Specificity was greater for:
- **Mammography (89.5%)**
- **Color Doppler (85.8%)**

Comparing the positive predictive value (PPV), the results were:
- **Physical examination (75%)**
- **Mammography (84%)**
- **Ultrasound (80%)**
- **Color Doppler (82%)**

And the negative predictive value (NPV):
- **Physical examination (82.1%)**
- **Mammography (89.5%)**
- **Ultrasound (96.8%)**
- **Color Doppler (94.3%)**

When the Bayes sequential test was used in this analysis there was a resultant increase in the PPV. This means that while color Doppler is useful in cases where the other diagnostic methods give positive results, it is even more useful in cases where some of the results are negative.

2) *Flow Rate: Indexes and Velocities*

Our experience in this area has been much like that of other researchers, and we have yet to find differences between the R.I. and the P.I. values significant enough to allow differential diagnoses between benign and malignant tumors.

Although it is true that in general these vessels show low resistance, ample diastole and high velocities, we do not use these indexes at this time.

However, we have found greater velocities in malignant tumors than in benign tumors, and the differences are significant. In these neoplasies the general velocity often exceeds 25 to 40 cm/s, speeds which rarely occur in benign tumors.

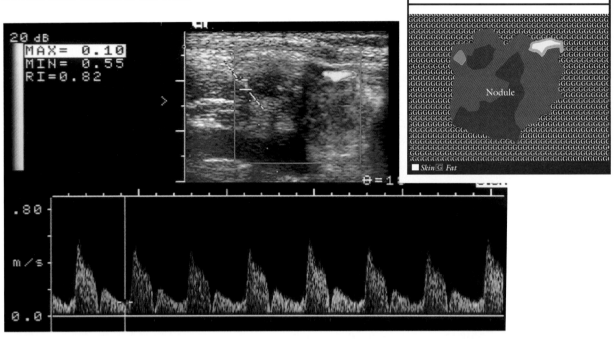

Fig. 14.27 Image of a supraclavicular lymph node with irregular borders, heterogeneous echoes, and two vascular poles. It was diagnosed as an infiltrating ductal carcinoma with ganglionar metastasis:
     M.S.V.: 10 cm/s
     M.D.V.: 08 cm/s

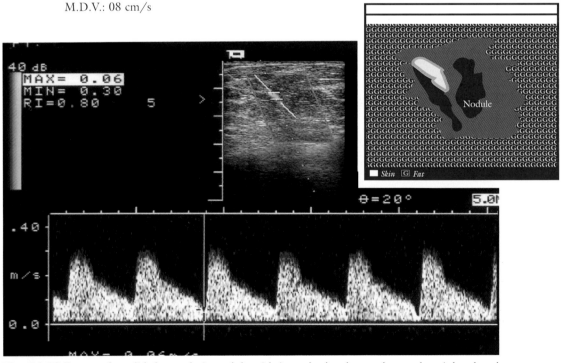

Fig. 14.28 Image of a solid, hypoechoic nodule with irregular borders and several peripheral and central vascular signals. Infiltrating ductal carcinoma. The image displays an elongated Color Doppler signal within the mass:
     M.S.V.: 30cm/s   M.D.V.: 06cm/s

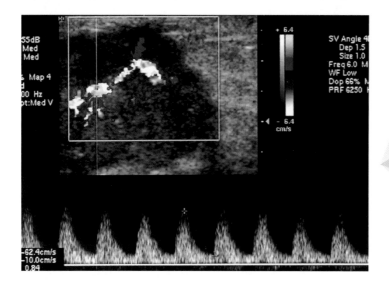

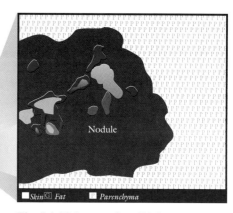

Fig. 14.29 Image of a solid, heterogeneous nodule which shows hypervascularization and mosaicism in one sector:
M.S.V.: 62.4 cm/s   R.I.: 0.84 cm/s

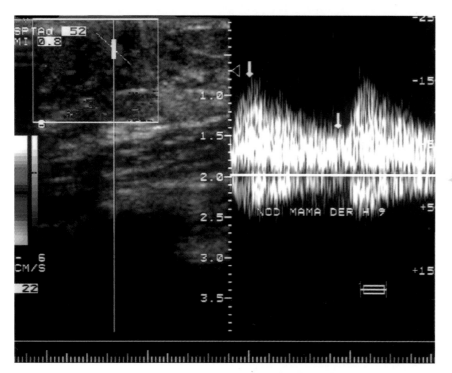

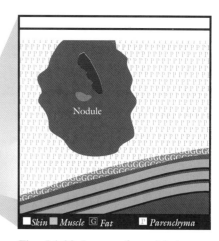

Fig. 14.30 Image of a solid, heterogeneous nodule with irregular borders and multiple interior and peripheral vascular signals. It was diagnosed as a carcinoma.

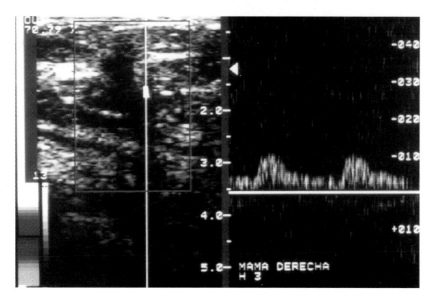

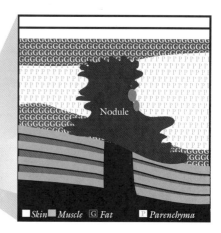

Fig. 14.31 Image of a solid nodule with completely irregular borders, sonic attenuation, and a dotted Color Doppler vascular signal in several sectors. Infiltrating ductal carcinoma.

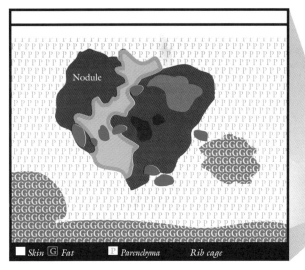

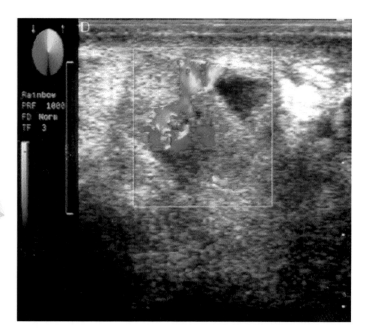

Fig. 14.32 Image of a nodule with heterogeneous echostructure and a focus of necrosis. There is a vascular signal occupying more than 30% of the tumor's volume; the vessels are tortuous, irregular, shunted, and located both inside and outside the nodule.

A study by Madyar in which the systolic velocities of all the vessels in a tumor were added resulted in the AMSV (addition of the maximum systolic velocities). It was found that the velocity associated with malignant tumors is 285 cm/s while that associated with benign tumors is 29 cm/s.

C. Sohn et al. use a technique called (MEM, maximum entropy method) to measure blood flow by ultrasound. This method allows the study of vessels with extremely low velocities which cannot be studied using conventional color Doppler. The minimum velocity which can be detected using this technique is 0.1 mm/s using a PRF: 210 Hz. Color Doppler, on the other hand, can detect velocities between 1 and 3 cm/s.

The image is divided into three types of signals:
- **An individual signal within a tumor.**
- **An area within the tumor.**
- **Several areas within the tumor.**

When comparing the results of ultrasound and MEM in benign tumors (N:71) and malignant tumors (N:121) the following percentages of correct diagnoses are produced:

	Benign tumor	**Malignant tumor**
B-mode exclusively	76.06%	83.47%
MEM exclusively	76.06%	89.26%
Mode B and MEM	90.14%	95.87%
Table 13.2		

MEM classifies tumors which have no blood flow or which have less than 5 pixels as benign. Tumors with more than 5 pixels or which show blood flow are classified as malignant.

In another study in which MEM was employed color Doppler was shown to be a valuable tool for prognosis because blood flow can be correlated with the size of the tumor, the ganglionar stage, the hormonal receptors, and ploidy and cell division in S-phase.

The study concludes that small tumors without ganglionar metastasis and with positive receptors, diploid genome, and low cell division in S-phase are the tumors with the lowest blood flow.

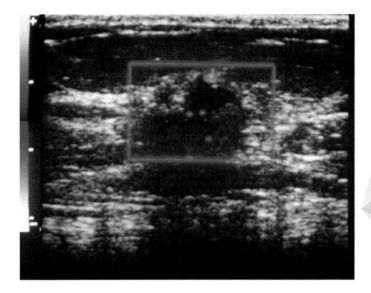

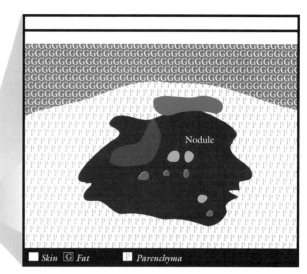

Fig. 14.33 Evaluation of a solid, malignant nodule in B MEM mode (image courtesy of Dr. C. Sohn).

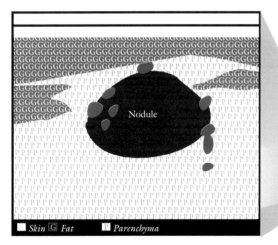

Fig. 14.34 Evaluation of a solid, benign nodule in B MEM mode (image courtesy of Dr. C. Sohn).

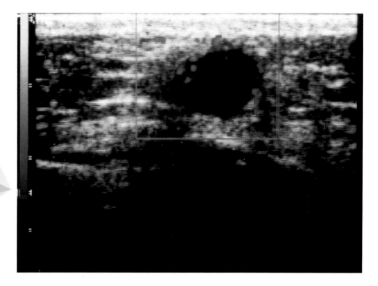

Another method for studying tumor vascularization is power Doppler, which measures the power of the Doppler signal, instead of the direction and velocity of blood flow. This method is effective in the hands of a trained technician; the main disadvange is that the patient's breathing can produce artifact. However, this can normally be overcome by adjusting the power gain. The most important difference between color Doppler and power Doppler is the ability of the latter to observe slow blood flows and very small vessels. Power Doppler is more successful at producing vascular images regardless of the angle employed or the tortuosity of the vessels.

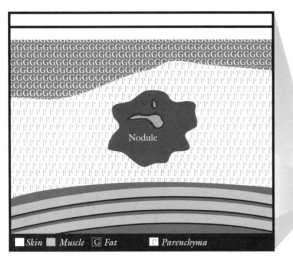 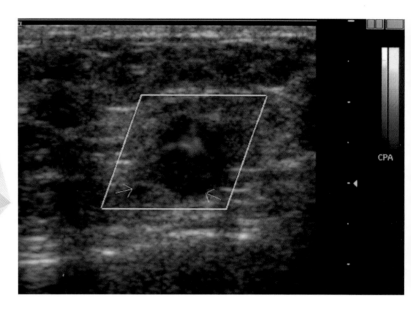

Skin ▪ Muscle G Fat P Parenchyma

Figs. 14.35, 14.36 Power Doppler images displaying a peripheral vascular ring and a large interior vessel.

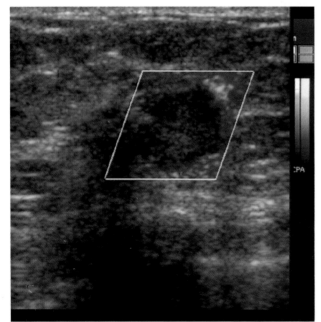 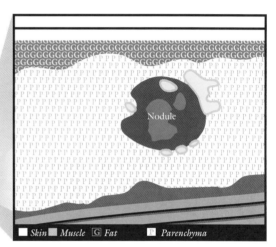

Skin ▪ Muscle G Fat P Parenchyma

Fig. 14.36 See above.

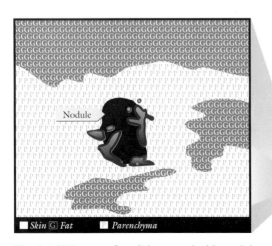 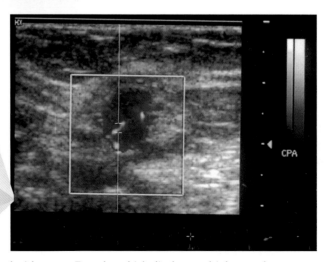

Skin G Fat P Parenchyma

Fig. 14.37 Image of a solid, non-palpable nodule explored with power Doppler which displays multiple vascular signals. It was diagnosed as a carcinoma.

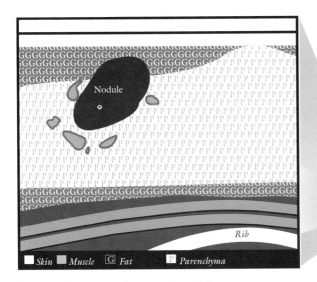

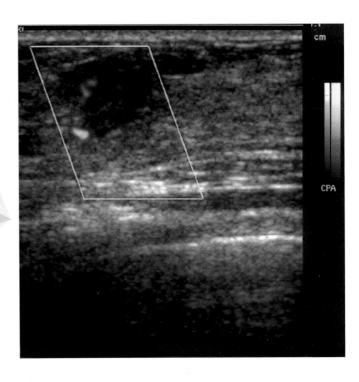

Fig. 14.38 Image of a nodule which appears benign; Power Doppler study shows a peripheral vascular signal and an absence of interior signals.

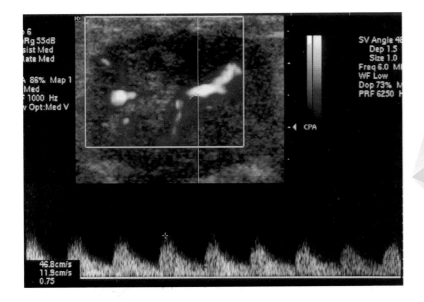

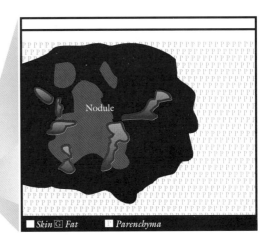

Fig. 14.39 Image of a tumor 38mm in size with defined borders, heterogeneous echostructure, and a significant central vascular signal when analyzed with power Doppler.

M.S.V.: 46.8 cm/s

D.V.: 11cm/s

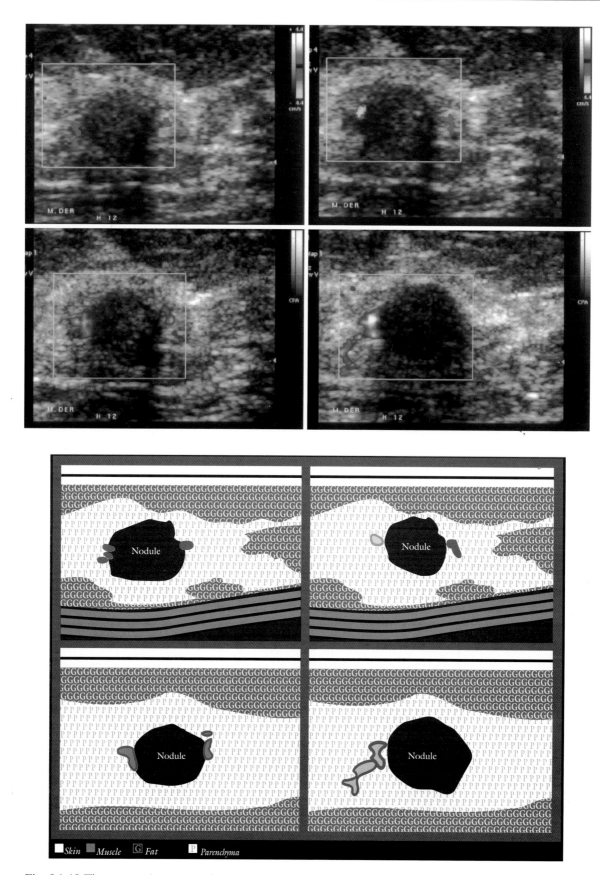

Fig. 14.40 The two top images are obtained with color Doppler images and the two bottom images with power Doppler. Both methods show a peripheral vascular signal. The nodule is a fibroadenoma.

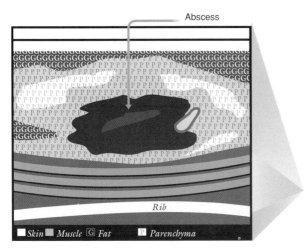

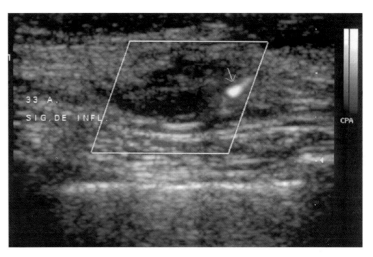

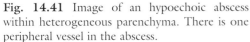

Fig. 14.41 Image of an hypoechoic abscess within heterogeneous parenchyma. There is one peripheral vessel in the abscess.

Dynamic Angiographic Ultrasound (DAU) 3-D

DAU 3-D is a new technology which employs power Doppler to produce a three-dimensional image of the vascularization of a mass or tumor. The image is dynamic, appears in real time, and allows observation of all areas of the mass in question.

DAU 3-D allows the storage in memory of up to eleven sequences of images, which are then assembled and appear on the screen as the mass itself in 3-D and rotating on an axis.

A map is also produced which aids in the quantification of the neovascularization, and the entire sequence can be recorded on videotape. This is a new technology and it must undergo further testing, but it is expected to become a very important tool for non-invasive diagnosis.

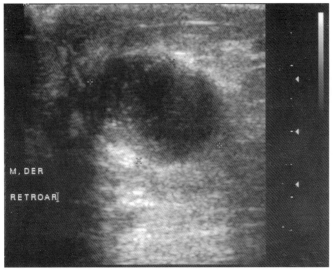

I.

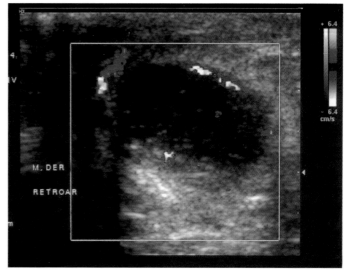

II.

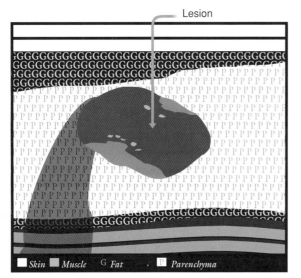

Fig. 14.42 Images showing various evaluation methods: **I.** Ultrasound in B mode image displays a hypoechoic nodule, 22 x 15mm in size, 10mm deep within the gland, which produces heterogeneous interior echoes and sonic attenuation in one sector. **II.** A color Doppler image of the same nodule displays two oblique and heterogeneous vascular trajectories and three 'spot' signals in other sectors. **III.** The power Doppler image of the same nodule shows an elongated, curved peripheral vascular trajectory in the posterior sector and a small signal in the anterior sector. **IV.** A second power Doppler image shows a curved vascular signal in the anterior sector and reveals other 'spot' signals in the posterior sector.

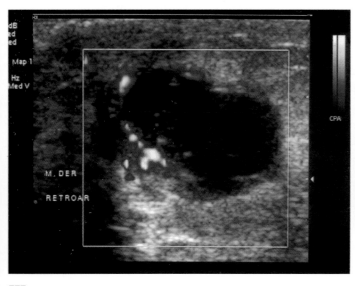

III.

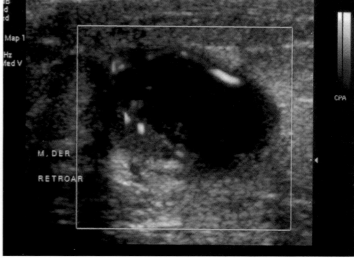

IV.

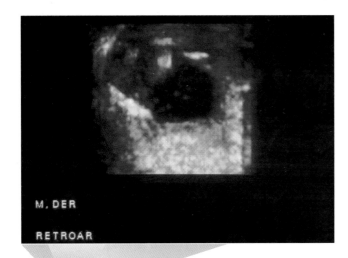 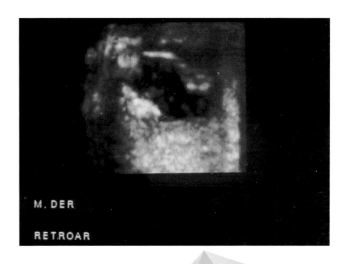

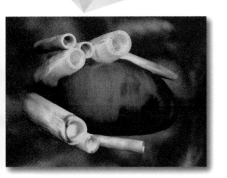 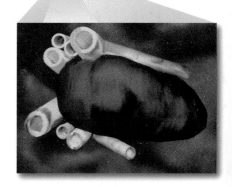

Fig. 14.43 The two images at top were taken in DAU 3-D as part of a sequence of 11 sections recorded on video. The images below demonstrate the rotation of the image possible with this system.

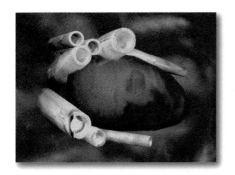 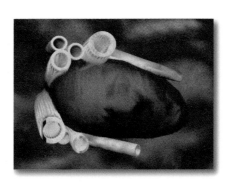 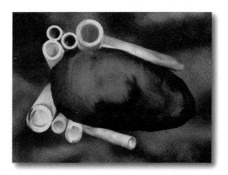

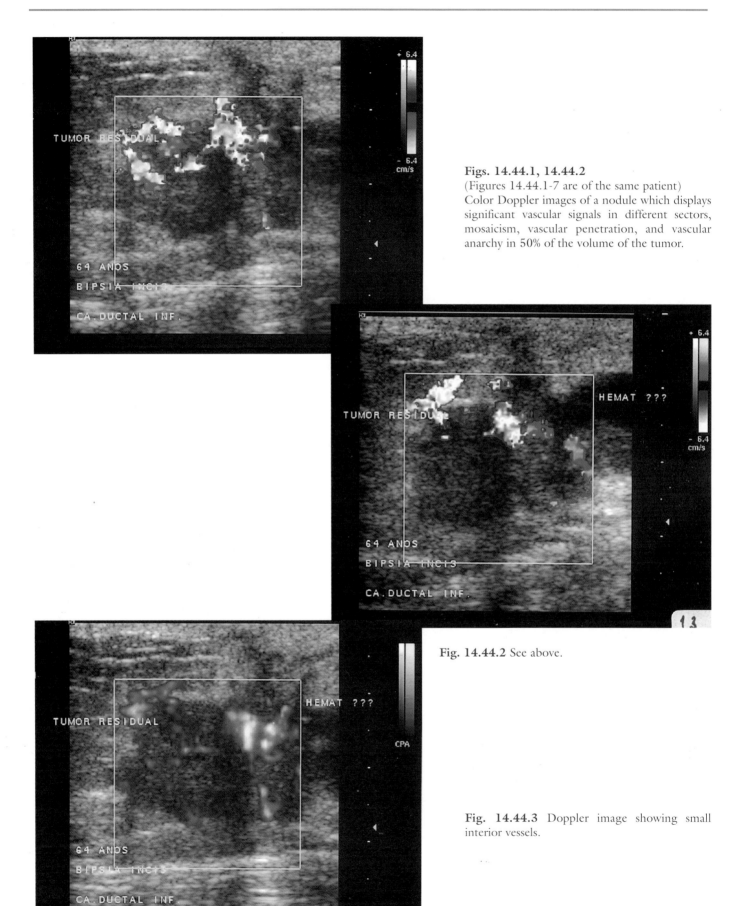

Figs. 14.44.1, 14.44.2
(Figures 14.44.1-7 are of the same patient)
Color Doppler images of a nodule which displays significant vascular signals in different sectors, mosaicism, vascular penetration, and vascular anarchy in 50% of the volume of the tumor.

Fig. 14.44.2 See above.

Fig. 14.44.3 Doppler image showing small interior vessels.

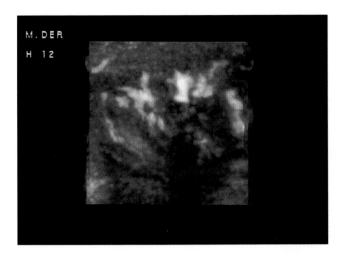

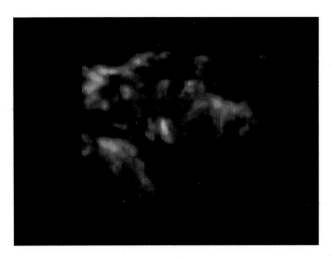

Figs. 14.44.4- 14.44.6 DAU 3-D images show tortuous vascular trajectories centrally and peripherally located and occupying 80% of the tumor.

Fig. 14.44.5

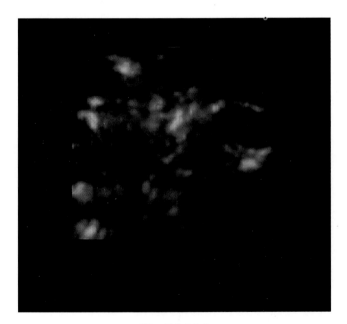

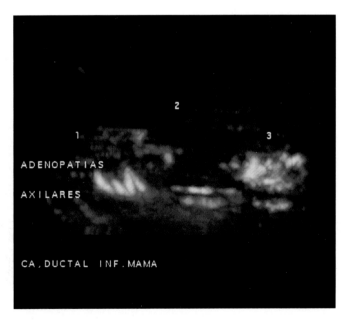

Fig. 14.44.6

Fig. 14.44.7 DAU 3-D image displaying 3 lymph nodes suspected of metastasis. It was diagnosed as an infiltrating ductal carcinoma with scarce differentiation, a high degree of anaplasia, a low mitotic rate, and vascular and lymph node invasion.

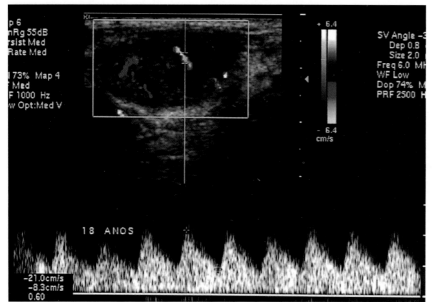
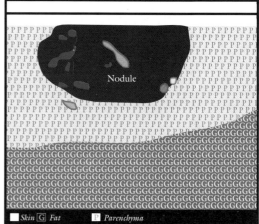

Fig. 14.45.1 Color Doppler image of a fibroadenoma in an 18 year-old patient displaying linear and 'spot' type vascular images in central and peripheral locations.

M.S.V.: 21 cm/s
D.V.: 8.3 cm/s
R.I.: 0.60

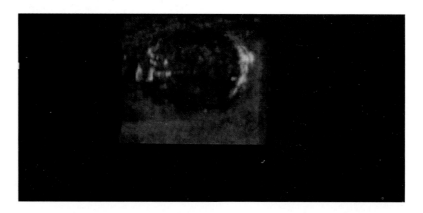

Fig. 14.45.2 DAU 3-D image of the patient in Fig. 14.45.1. showing a predominantly peripheral vascular signal.

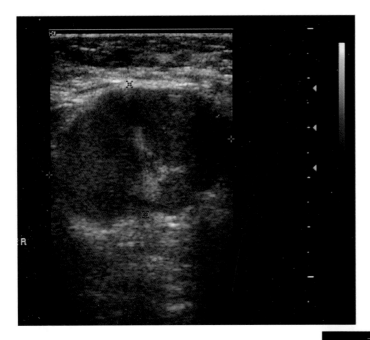

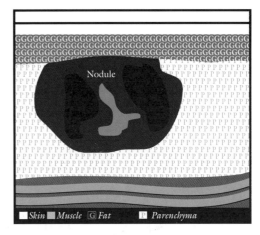

Fig. 14.46.1 (Figures 14.46.1-3 are of the same patient) Image of a solid, polilobulated nodule with defined borders and heterogeneous echostructure, 38 x26mm in size in a 33 year-old patient complaining of a palpable nodule in the upper-outer quadrant of the right breast.

Fig. 14.46.2 Color Doppler image shows an internal vascular system which occupies 90% of the tumor and displays shunts, mosaicism and vascular anarchy.

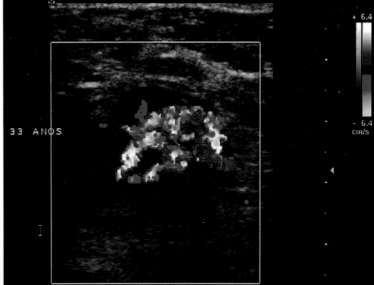

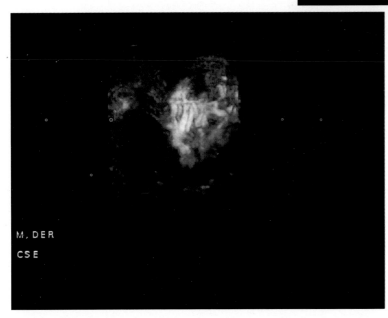

Fig. 14.46.3 DAU 3-D image displays all vascular trajectories. An infiltrating ductal carcinoma was diagnosed by biopsy, with 10 lymph nodes affected by areas of lobular carcinoma and metastasis.

Lymph Node Evaluation with Color Doppler

The evaluation of the axillary lymph nodes is fundamental in prognosis and the planning of treatment, and the use of this method has been studied extensively. Statistics show that the sensitivity in the detection of metastasis of the axillary lymph nodes is between 82 and 84%; specificity is between 90 and 95%; the positive predictive value is approximately 92%.

Metastasis detection can be improved if the vascular patterns are analyzed; Walsh et al. have applied similar techniques to the study of adenopathies and have obtained the following results:

- **Sensitivity: 70%**
- **Specificity: 98%**
- **PPV: 96%**

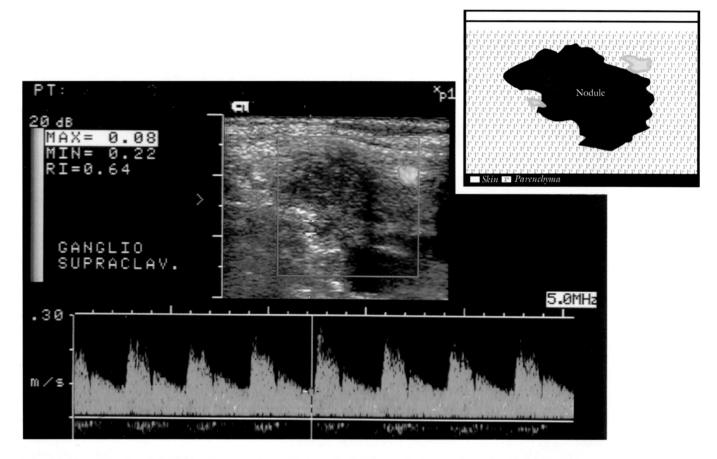

Fig. 14.47 Image of a solid, heterogeneous nodule with irregular borders and two vascular poles: A ductal carcinoma with lymph node metastasis was diagnosed:

M.S.V.: 45 cm/s
M.D.V.: 10 cm/s

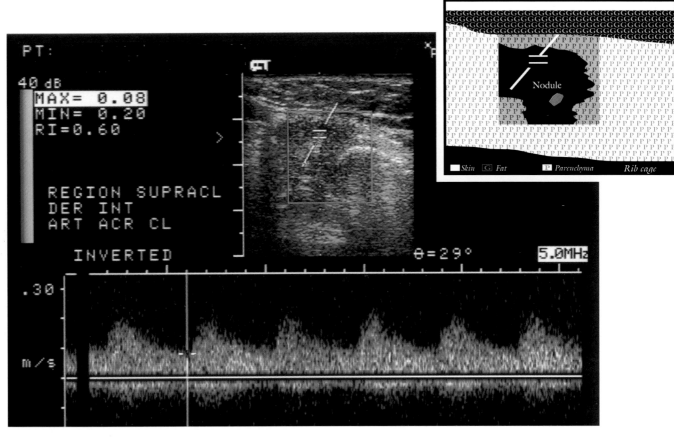

Figs. 14.48, 14.49 Images of a patient with a prior surgery for breast carcinoma referred for a palpable supraclavicular adenopathy. Using Color Doppler the nodule appears small, heterogeneous and hypoechoic. A metastasis from carcinoma was diagnosed:

M.S.V.: 20 cm/s
M.D.V.: 10 cm/s

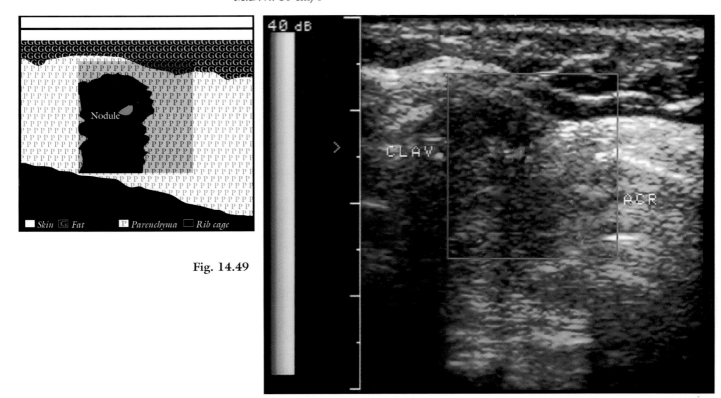

Fig. 14.49

Breast Ultrasound

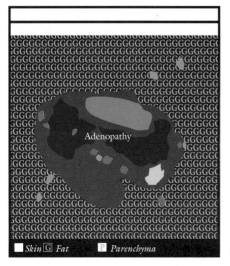

Fig. 14.50 Image of metastasis in a patient with a history of breast cancer; the nodule is a heterogeneous axillary adenopathy with irregular borders and multiple vascular signals.

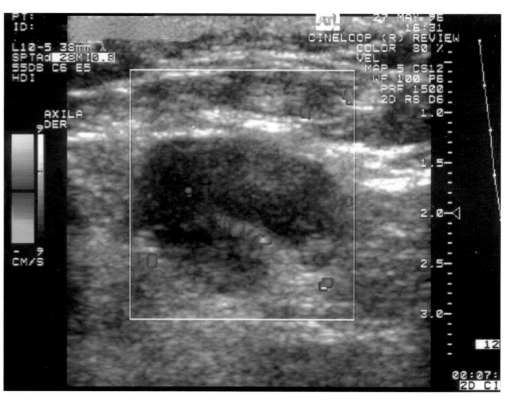

The risk of metastasis in tumors larger than 1 cm is approximately 30%; in non-palpable tumors not smaller than 1 cm it is between 15 and 20%; however, the percentage increases to 70% or more if the tumor reaches stage III.

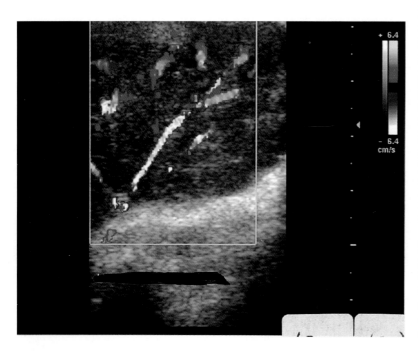

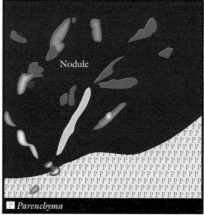

Fig. 14.51.1
(Figures 14.51.1-2 are of the same patient)
Color Doppler image of a nodule in a 30 year-old patient complaining of a palpable tumor on the axillary tail of the left breast. The mass contacts the skin and is solid with smooth borders, heterogeneous echostructure and a series of lineal vessels creating a mosaicism.

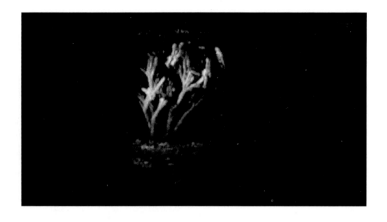

Fig. 14.51.2 A DAU 3-D image which shows lineal vessels which occupy 60-70% of the tumor. Biopsy confirmed a systemic lymph node pathology, possibly of lymphomatose origin.

Prognostic Possibilities

Doppler technology allows the radiologist to analyze and quantify a tumor and establish a prognostic value linked to the agressiveness of the tumor, its growth rate, and its potential for developing metastasis.

Hypervascularization in a tumor can be classified as grade III agressiveness. This means:

- **The percentage of vascularization may be used as an index for the agressiveness and the rate of evolution of the tumor.**

- **One can determine the success of auxillary treatments by the increase or decrease in vascularization.**

Sohn et al. conducted a study using color Doppler and MEM in 157 patients with invasive ductal carcinomas. The use of these combined technologies allowed the detection of slow blood flows. The majority of the cases with low blood flow were cases of small tumors, with positive hormonal receptors and without ganglionar metastasis. The majority of the tumors with aneuploid genomes showed increased vascularization per pixel or per area.

The detection of estrogen and progesterone receptors correlates with low levels of vascularization, while lack of these receptors correlates with high levels of vascularization. Tumoral vessels are low-resistance vessels with low velocity flows, due to the lack of a muscular layer in their walls.

Although further studies are necessary, these analyses may become an important part of pre-surgical prognosis.

99% of malignant tumors have three or more vessels, and 75% have five or more. Even considering the limitations of color Doppler (changes in the color and caliber of vessels) and the tortuosity of vascular systems, 75 to 80% of malignant tumors are diagnosed using this system.

Yet another prognostic possibility has to do with patients who have been diagnosed by cytological or histological puncture as having cancer and are undergoing auxillary therapies prior to radiology or surgery. In these cases a study should be performed prior to and after treatment. These studies will yield one of three results:

1) **A negative response, with progression of the disease and lack of vascular alteration.**

2) **A complete response, with disappearance of the tumor, lack of metastasis, and a disappearance of the vascular signal.**

3) **A partial response, with a 50% decrease in tumor size, and a decrease in metastasis.**

In cases in which vascularization decreases, a subsequent decrease in the size of the tumor will be observed.

Color Doppler is especially useful in cases in which clinical examination is difficult due to diffuse or very soft tumors, or tumors which seem to increase in size due to areas of necrosis or hemorrhage. It is also useful in cases in which the size of the tumor cannot be determined by B mode due to sonic attenuation, or because the tumor exceeds the diameter of the transducer.

Evaluation of Auxillary Treatments

In a study conducted in 1994 Cosgrove et al. observed 34 patients with large or centrally-located breast tumors. These patients could not undergo surgery and were scheduled for chemotherapy. Two evaluations were performed on each patient with both color Doppler and ultrasound in B mode. Patients were examined before and after treatment in order to observe their responses to chemotherapy. It was found that changes in vascularization matched changes in tumor size, i.e. a decrease in vascularization was accompanied by a decrease in tumor size. However, the most interesting finding was that changes in vascularization were observable by color Doppler approximately 4 weeks before changes in tumor size were noted by clinical or ultrasound examinations. From these findings Cosgrove et al. concluded that color Doppler can be used to predict response to chemotherapy.

Angiostatic Agents

In addition to commonly used antineoplastic drugs, a number of substances which inhibit angiogenesis are being investigated. Studies by J. Folkman demonstrate the important role that angiogenesis plays in tumor growth and evolution. Numerous studies exist which support Folkman's findings and current studies are being performed *in vitro* and on animals with substances which stimulate or inhibit angiogenesis.

There are nine stimulating factors, six of which are growth factors:

- **Fibroblastic growth factor**
- **Vascular endothelial placentary factor**
- **Transformation factor**
- **Hepatocytic factor**
- **Factor from cells derived from platelets**
- **Angiogenin**
- **Interleukin-8**
- **Granulocytic factor I**
- **Granulocytic factor II**

There are also nine inhibiting factors:

- **Factor 4**
- **Fumagilin (derived from TNP-470)**
- **Plaquetary**
- **Interleukin-12**
- **Metaloproteinase inhibitor**
- **Carboxiaminotriasol**
- **Talidomide**
- **Interferon alpha 2A**
- **Linomide**
- **Polysaccharide sulfate tecogalianide (DS-4152)**

Research indicates that the process of vascularization is controlled by an equilibrium between inhibiting and stimulating factors. Preliminary studies also indicate that angiostatic factors may be more effective when combined with chemotherapeutic cytotoxins.

Contrast Agents

Contrast agents, also known as signal enhancers, are used to aid diagnosis in patients with previous non-conclusive examinations. Used in breast examinations, these agents can aid in the early detection of tumors and in the identification of neoplasias. Signal enhancers increase the echogenic contrast. These substances were originally used in the evaluation of cardiac images, but their use has now spread to other areas.

Signal enhancers are delivered intravenously; they do not produce side effects and they remain stable long enough for an examination to be performed. The agent used in breast tumors was initially designated SHU-508; it is composed of gas-filled microbubbles suspended in water and stabilized with palmitic acid and galactose microparticles.

Ultrasound waves cause tissues to vibrate at the same frequency as the stimulus, and thus they produce heat. Ultrasound waves applied to microbubbles induce vibrations and rhythmic compression and expansion. The vibrations and the rhythmic expansion and contraction induce both harmonic and oscillation frequencies.

Signal enhancers have been approved by the FDA for use on animals, and Italy, Germany and Great Britain have approved the substance for clinical application on humans. A study conducted involving 2,403 patients revealed no side-effects except for some cases of local pain and irritation. Breakdown of SHU-508 occurs in the liver by an insulin-independent mechanism, and half-life in a healthy adult is 10-11 minutes.

Clinical efficiency in the breast was demonstrated in a study on ninety-one patients in four different clinics. The following results were obtained:

Diagnostic reliability prior to injection:
40 +/- 24 %
Diagnostic reliability after injection: 73 +/- 18 %
Variation in the diagnosis: 97 %

SHU-508 does not seem to produce many changes in the images of benign tumors. However, when used in cases of malignant tumors it makes the detection of vessels much easier and information such as the number of vessels, their tortuosity, and the number of shunts is much more easily obtained.

The future for color Doppler in the field of breast examinations is very promising. Color Doppler allows one to observe and analyze the vascular structures, location, and exact characteristics of a tumor and arrive at a prognosis.

One can determine the characteristics of a tumor with ultrasound in B mode with 85-90% accuracy; the ability to analyze blood flow to the tumor further increases diagnostic precision and accuracy, as blood flow is positively correlated with malignancy.

Color Doppler is non-invasive and particularly useful in cases in which ultrasound in B mode is inconclusive, where scar tissues produce sonic attenuation, and in the follow-up after conservative breast surgery.

The rapid advances in the field of ultrasound raise a number of questions: will the number of surgeries performed decrease as a result of the increased ability to determine if a tumor is benign or malignant? And how will the information provided by new technologies affect surgical techniques?

What will the future hold? Perhaps ultrasonic tumor therapy will be possible, destroying the blood vessels of the tumor with a direct beam of ultrasound. Another possibility is the use of microbubbles filled with angiostatic chemicals which burst upon demand in the location where they are most needed.

Concerning angiogenesis: can it be controlled by means of drug therapy? Current studies in this field are hoped to provide an answer to this question soon.

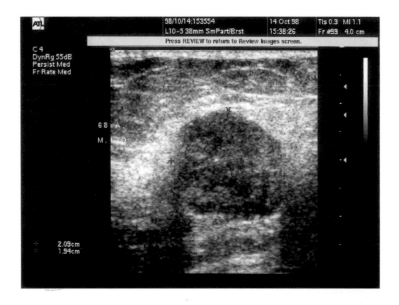

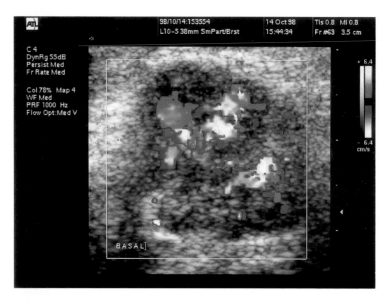

Fig. 14.52 Images of a solid nodule with poorly-defined borders, partial sonic attenuation, and heterogeneous echostructure. Prior to injection of contrast agent the vascular signal is weak, but it improves significantly after the injection .

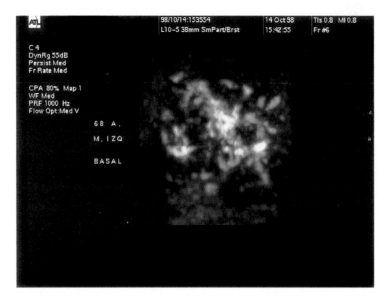

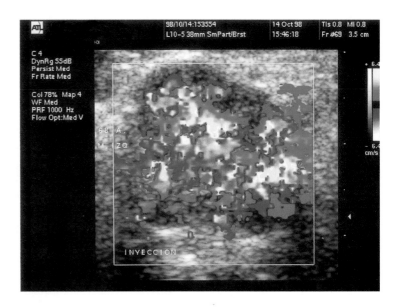

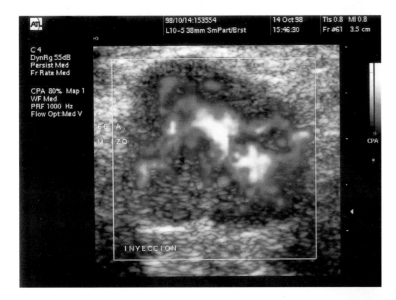

Fig. 14.53 Images of a solid, bilobulated nodule with defined borders and a small calcification. Only one vessel is detected before injection of contrast agent but after injection several vascular signals were detected.

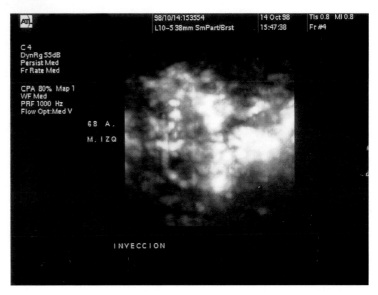

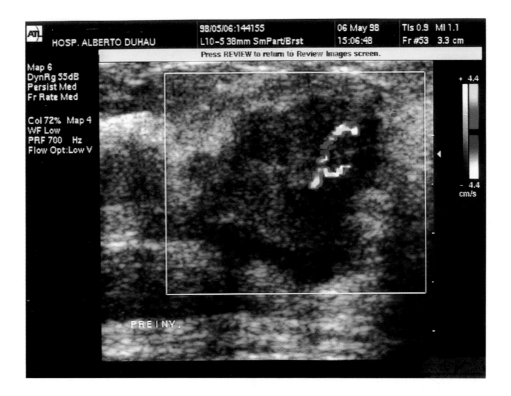

Fig. 14.54 (Figures 14.54-15.60 are of the same patient)
Color Doppler image of a solid nodule with irregular borders and heterogeneous echostructure which displays a bifurcated vascular signal in one sector.

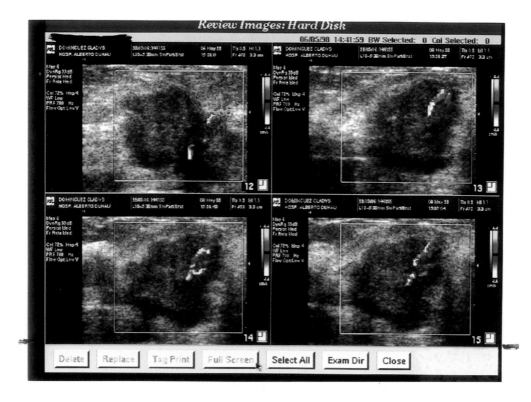

Fig. 14.55 Various images of the tumor which show low levels of basal vascularization.

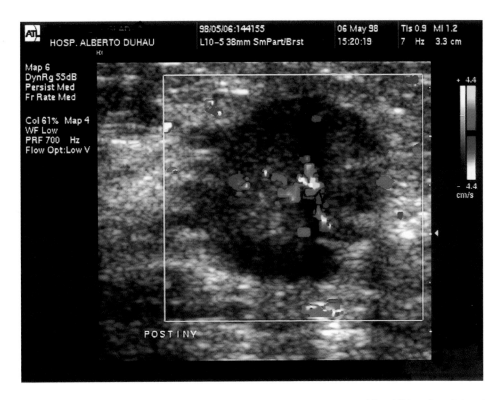

Fig. 14.56 After injection of a contrast agent the image is improved by 40% and peripheral vessels become visible.

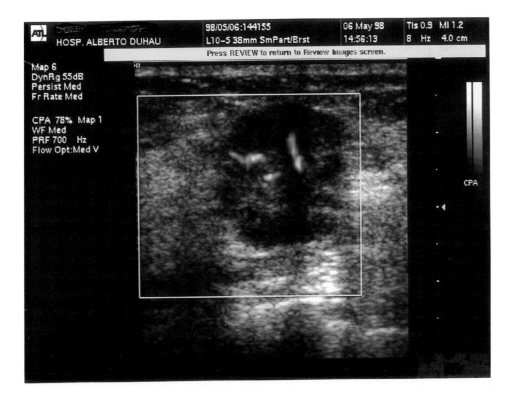

Fig. 14.57 Doppler Power image of the same tumor shows three centrally-located lineal vessels and a weak peripheral signal.

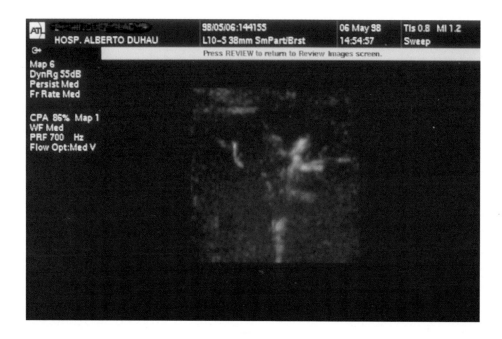

Fig. 14.58 After injection of a contrast agent the Doppler signal appears stronger and visualization of the vessels is improved 40-60%.

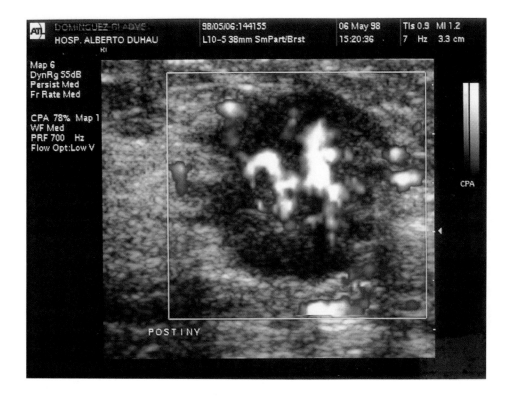

Fig. 14.59 DAU 3-D image of the tumor showing a vessel in front of the tumor, discrete bifurcation to the right, and a lineal signal to the left.

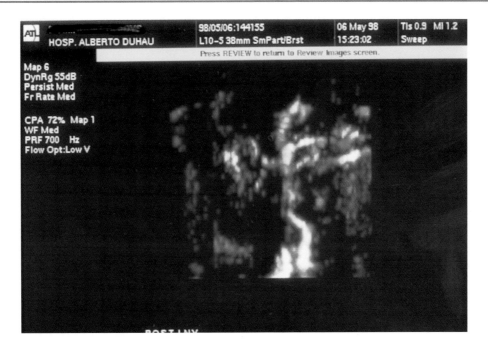

Fig. 14.60 After the Levoist injection and using DAU 3-D the strength of the signal and number of vessels seen are increased 60-70%.

References

- Dock W: Tumor Vascularization: Assessment with Duplex Sonography. *Radiology,* 1991; 181:241-244.
- Adler DD, Carson PL, Rubin JM, Quinn Reid D: Doppler Ultrasound Color Flow Imaging in the Study of Breast Cancer: Preliminary Findings. *Ultrasound Med Biol,* 1990, 16:553-559.
- Cosgrove, JC, Bamber, JB, Davey *et al.*: Color Doppler signals from Breast Tumors. *Radiology* 1990; 176:175-180.
- Burns PN, Davies JD, Halliwell M, *et al.*: Doppler Ultrasound in the Diagnostis of Breast Cancer. In: *Ultrasound in Breast and Endocrine Disease-Clinics in Diagnostic Ultrasound* (12), edited by GR Leopold, Churchil Livingstone, New York, 1984, pp. 41-56.
- Cosgrove JC, Bamber JB, Davey *et al.*: Color Doppler Signals from Breast Tumours, Work in Progress. *Radiology* 1990; 176: 175-180.
- Madjar H, Vetter M, Prompeler HJ, Wieacker P, Schillinger H.: The Normal Vascularization of the Female Breast in Doppler Ultrasound. *Ultraschall- Med.,* 1992 Aug, 13 (4): 171-177.
- Sohn C, Grischke EM, Wallwiener D, Kaufmann M, von Fournier D, Bastert G: Ultrasound Diagnosis of Blood Flow in Benign and Malignant Breast Tumors. *Geburtshilfe Frauenheilkd.* 1992, Jul; 52 (7):397-403.
- Luska G, Lott D, Risch U, von Boetticher H: The Findings of Color Doppler Sonography in Breast Tumors. Rofo, Fortschr, Geb, Rontgenstr, Neuen, Bildgeb, Verfahr, 1992, Feb, 156 (2):142-5.
- Madjar H, Prompeler H, Schurmann R, Goppinger A, Breckwoldt M, Pfleiderer A: Improving Diagnosis of Breast Tumors by Echo-Contrast Media. Geburtshilfe, Frauenheilkd, 1993, Dec; 53 (12): 866-9.
- Cosgrove DO, Kedar RP, Bamber JC, Murrani B, Davey JB, Fisher C, McKinna JA, Svensson WE, Tohno E, Vagios E, *et al.*: Breast Diseases: Color Doppler US in Differential Diagnosis. *Radiology,* 1993, Oct; 189 (1):99-104.
- Bergonzy M, Calliada F, Corsi G, Passamonti C, Bonfioli C, Motta F, Urani A: Role of Echo-Color Doppler in the Diagnosis of Breast Diseases. *Radiol Med Torino,* 1993, May; 85 (5 Suppl. 1):120-123.
- Spreafico C, Lanocita R, Frigerio LF, Di Tolla G, Garbagnati F, Milella M, Marchiano A, Piragine G, Damascelli: The Italian Experience with SH U 508 A (Levovist) in Breast Disease. *Radiol Med-Torino.* 1994, May; 87 (5 suppl. 1): 59-64.
- Walsh JS, Dixon JM, Chetty U, Paterson D: Color Doppler Studies of Axillary Node Metastases in Breast Carcinoma. *Clin- Radiol,* 1994, Mar; 49 (3):189-91.
- Calliada F, Raieli G, Sala G, Conti MP, Bottinelli O, La Fianza A, Bergonzi M, Campani R: Doppler Color Echo in the Sonographic Evaluation of Solid Neoplasms of the Breast. *Radiol-Med Torino.* 1994, Jan-Feb; 87 (1-2): 28-35.
- Shon C, Krunes U, Becker D, Gunter E, Mutze S, Steinkamp W Muller, Westkott HP, Gebel M: Possibilities and Limits of a New Color Technique Ultrasound Angiography. *Bildgebung.* 1995, Mar; 62 (1):53-63.
- Lagalla R, Caruso G, Marasa L, D' Angelo I, Cardinale AE: Angiogenic Capacity of Breast Neoplasms and Correlation with Color Doppler Semiology. *Radiol Med Torino.* 1994, Oct; 88 (4): 392-395.
- Mirta Ester Lanfranchi, Norman Ignacio Koremblit: Terapia ultrasónica tumoral (TUT): *Revista Argentina de Radiología.* vol. 59, nº 2, 1995; 127-129.

15

Three-Dimensional Ultrasound

M. E. Lanfranchi

Three-dimensional ultrasound (3DUS) is a new and promising technology which dramatically increases the diagnostic capability of sonography by providing the ultrasound technologist an image in three dimensions which can be manipulated so as to allow the visualization of an area of interest from a number of different angles.

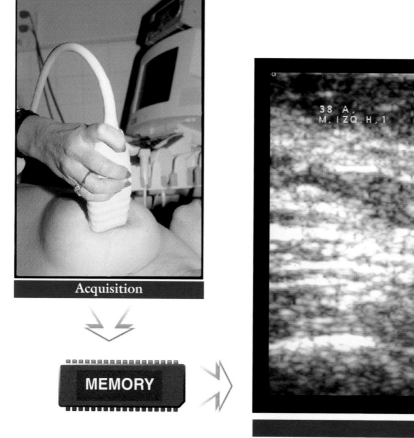

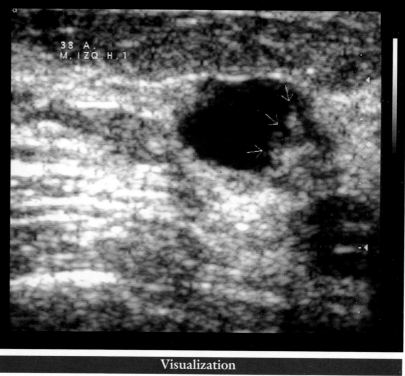

Figure 15.1 Acquisition and visualization of ultrasound images.

Acquisition

Two-dimensional ultrasound (2DUS) emits and receives ultrasound beams along a single two-dimensional plane providing a single tomographical section of an object. 3DUS, on the other hand, emits beams along numerous adjacent planes and stores each section in memory. The numerous sections acquired by 3DUS provide information on depth and volume, and the ability to store information in memory allows one to select and combine sections.

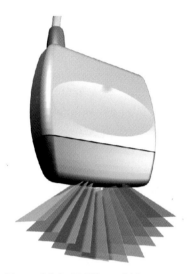

Figure 15.2 3DUS acquisition.

Visualization

2DUS offers visualization of only one plane (see figure 15.3 below). 3DUS acquires and stores in memory a number of different views of the area of interest. In addition to the longitudinal and sagittal sections which

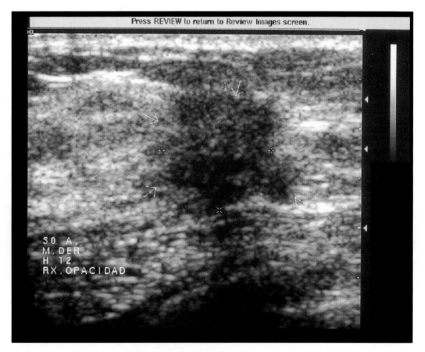

Figure 15.3 2DUS visualization.

2DUS can provide, 3DUS offers a coronal (frontal) view. The information stored in memory can be presented in two ways, the simultaneous display of multiple sections or the reconstruction of the area of interest in three dimensions.

Figure 15.3 below demonstrates the simultaneous display of multiple sections.

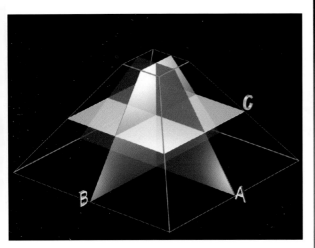

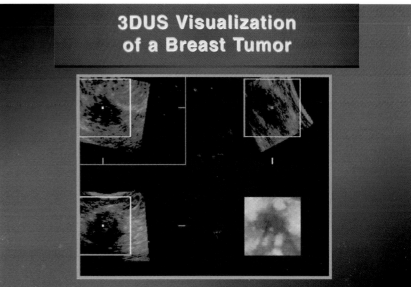

Figure 15.4 Multiple Sections; A: longitudinal, B: sagittal, C: coronal.

Improvements in computer technology allow workstations to carry out the complex algorithms necessary to add volume to sections acquired by ultrasound, providing a view of an object in its standard anatomical orientation and in three dimensions (see fig. 15.4 below).

To date few articles have been published concerning the application of 3DUS to breast examination, but there is little doubt that this technology will aid tremendously in the diagnosis of breast pathologies by ultrasound.

Figure 15.4 Three-dimensional reconstruction. *(Image courtesy of MEDISON).*

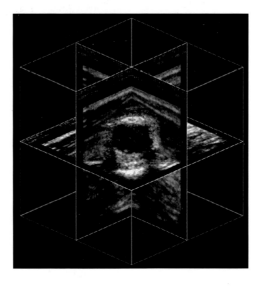